A Difficult Time

A Difficult Time

My Journey in Medicine

Jerry Sobieraj, M.D.

Writer's Showcase
San Jose New York Lincoln Shanghai

A Difficult Time
My Journey in Medicine

Writer's Showcase
an imprint of iUniverse, Inc.

For information address:
iUniverse, Inc.
5220 S. 16th St., Suite 200
Lincoln, NE 68512
www.iuniverse.com

ISBN: 0-595-20481-3

Printed in the United States of America

To Jan, Stephie and Jocie,
who helped me during my difficult time.

*Thanks to Jan and Chris for their thoughtful
review of this manuscript.*

Introduction

A difficult time, indeed! Changing my career wasn't a decision I took lightly. In fact, it wasn't a decision I made quickly either. My initial attempt to modify my career wasn't focused on any particular change, and turned out to be quite unfruitful. However, the continued perils of practicing Medicine prevented me from ignoring a change altogether. Finally after additional deliberate consideration, early in the year 2000, I was able to formulate and begin to execute a detailed plan as to how I would leave Medicine.

To me, a career implied durability with the potential to accumulate experience. The career I had chosen, Medicine, required extensive training. This led to a significant time lag before I could actually practice my trade. Yet, if I did not change careers, I felt as if I would have been held hostage to the folly of my youth. A decision I made when I was young (i.e. mid-20s), no longer seemed relevant to me. There was a confluence of societal factors which had made mid-life career changes less unusual, so it did not feel inappropriate to make this change. In fact, for many, industry no longer seemed interested in providing long term security, and with this change, employees had made a commensurate change in their expectation of longevity in the workplace. As a result, we the employed, had developed a greater willingness to change jobs, both within our fields, and outside of them.

Yet another important factor in my wanting a career change seemed more internal. There was disquiet in my soul. I had been asked by friends and family if it was a depressed mood which was the source of my disquietude. I am not religious, so I am not referring to a soul in this context, out of my spiritual being. That part of us which seems to be coming from our brain, but as we contemplate its existence, the less certain we are of our spirits origin. Those of us who came of age in the 1960s and early 1970s developed an expectation that we would be true to ourselves (unlike Vietnam and Nixon). Rather than live the forced life-style we inherited from the post-war 1950s, we decided to try and be honest with ourselves. To me, this implied a pervasive honesty, not a selective one. When I looked at my soul, I realized my time in Medicine had led to a conflict at my core being.

Thus, an evolution of external and internal factors had come into conflict by the time I reached my mid-career. Many of the difficulties I experienced in my practice every day made me feel uncomfortable with the many practical decisions I was making on behalf of my patients. As a result, I needed to resolve this conflict, and resolve it definitively if I were to remain true to my soul. Most days, the career I had chosen no longer seemed appropriate for me. The factors that attracted me to Medicine were no longer discernible in my daily life. Instead I was confronted with a routine, unchanging process. I longed to be rid of these doldrums, returning to the environs of my loved ones. My home came to take precedence. What was the point of this continued procession to the office when it was so meaningless, and filled with little, if any, excitement and anticipation?

These were the seeds of my career change. Yet, just as the Southern States did not attempt to secede from the Union without due consideration, I also required a reflective process to be certain that a career change would solve the problem. Before considering a career change, I had made attempts over several years to restructure my interests within Medicine. I worked as the Director of Health Services in a local public school system, and became quite interested in School Health. Yet school systems in Massachusetts weren't ready to make the investment recommended by the Centers for Disease Control and Prevention (CDC). I also worked on curriculum development, and saw a couple of promising areas of clinical research that could be quite useful in caring for patients. Yet, ultimately, I had the problem of insufficient time to make the investment necessary to attain the requisite skills to make a lateral move. This lack of time could also have been enough of a barrier to prevent a career change from ever happening (as it often does). Over time, I came to the realization that a significant and professionally satisfactory change would require a substantial effort on my part (not to mention the impact on my family). So, if the investment was going to be so great in the first place, why limit myself to Medicine? I began to consider the prospect of learning a new skill set. If I was going to invest the time to garner new skills, I wouldn't limit myself to my current field. I finally took a look at the big picture, and assessed other skills I had. How could these skills be utilized, and how could I develop them further?

The changes in the practice of Medicine had outpaced me. It occurred to me that I was called to a new profession, one included under the rubric of high tech, specifically, Information Technology (IT). This field barely existed in the late 1970s when I became hooked on cellular and molecular biology. What had kept me in the clinical (as opposed to research) realm of Medicine was my ability to effectively communicate with people. Ultimately, the time demands of this realm, and my inability to control these demands, stifled me. When I was asked by friends and acquaintances about work, I would mention my intentions to seek a new career in IT. Generally, they would raise the onus thrust upon doctors by HMOs and managed care. Yet, the reality was, HMOs and managed care had created order in some ways, but hindered health care delivery in other ways. Despite their flaws, HMOs alone were not the sole culprits. In this book, I have detailed many of the factors which have contributed to my dismay with Medicine. Some of them were likely longstanding, and only became known to me due to my submersion in primary care medicine. Others had been part of the evolution of the health care system. The health care system had changed in front of me, and what I saw, I couldn't continue to support, tacitly, nor explicitly.

This is the prelude to the story of my journey in Medicine, from my initial spark of curiosity, to my final undoing in primary care medicine. A journey that began with promise, but ended in dismay. Since I worked in an academic medical center, I had the opportunity to discuss many of the issues affecting primary care with people who were still in the midst of their training as physicians (i.e. residents). Most of them were hard working, and dedicated to the task at hand. I've always found this laudable. Yet, as a society, to transform Medicine once again into a career with longevity, we would need to act on the issues I have discussed in this book. At times I have told trainees, with all sincerity, that "Medicine is a good 20 year career". I said this not with anger or malice (but maybe with some disappointment). I said it from the perspective that I had learned a lot during my 20 years in the field. It did not feel wasted. I sensed that the knowledge and experience I had gained during this time would remain useful to me, yet in what way, I did not know.

As a final introductory note, I want to make the record perfectly clear. Some of the people and institutions I have portrayed might be viewed in a negative light. However, no portrayal was intended with malice nor ill will. The intention of this book has been to indicate how I have viewed my journey in the field of Medicine. Since I have not viewed all things in my life as positive, I have appropriately reflected that in this book. Now, to begin the journey through that difficult time!

Contents

Chapter 1

The Sunday Globe

Painstakingly, slowly, I turned the pages. The urge to scratch my nose felt strong, but I couldn't bear to see those dreaded ink smudges on my face. The bigger the newspaper, the more ink I'd get on my hands. Since I was reading the Sunday (Boston) Globe, which was always big, the ink was particularly problematic. Big also meant in this case, that it was filled with a large Classified Section. That, of course, was the point. I generally didn't read the paper to get news, for that, I preferred to listen to the radio. But I wasn't interested in news. I wanted the largest Want Ads section possible (I wasn't on line yet, and hadn't heard of jobs.com, the Monster Board, etc.).

After I set the paper down, I rinsed my hands and sat down quietly. I couldn't believe I felt the need to peruse the Sunday Classifieds. Yet, the thought of continuing on in Medicine for another month, let alone another year, seemed unbearable. Going to and from work hundreds of more times was too much to countenance.

Yet, how could this happen? I had believed my career in Medicine would be interminable only a decade ago; now it all appeared for naught. It wished I could "declare victory and go home", as Bob Dole had done during his tenure as Senate Majority Leader. Instead, it was time to declare defeat and look at other options. That was my reality.

The Want Ads were not very inviting. Though some ads appeared to be a good potential fit, when I decided to answer them, not much happened. Often I wouldn't hear back, and would begin to wonder, "Did my letter get lost in the mail?". Most of my rejections were in the form of no response. When I was ignored it was hard to know where I stood in the eyes of prospective employers. I had a lot of education and had acquired many skills, yet none of this seemed marketable.

The few responses I did get were not particularly encouraging. They would tell me my CV (curriculum vitae, which is Latin for resume) looked great, but not quite what they had in mind. Well, when I read the ad it sure made me feel I was appropriate for the position (at least enough to take the time to write a letter). What happened? Why didn't anyone want to hire me? I surmised this was the result when one tried to transfer one's skill set to what seemed like a reasonable alternative (e.g. consultant, health educator, etc.)

I had believed that becoming a physician wasn't just a job, but a career, a lifetime of growth and opportunity. Yet my inability to shift to a new career in the health care industry made me feel about as bottled up as an older person who hadn't had a bowel movement in a couple days, and didn't know what to do next to get things moving. What was I supposed to do? Sure, I had letters after my name. Yet outside the medical marketplace, I was an entry level 'commodity'. I felt that if I had applied to McDonald's the next day, I would have been put on the grill.

I've been asked, as have most physicians nowadays, "Would you do it all over again?". I have thought back to my interest and zeal of youth, and didn't see how I could have ended up elsewhere. Maybe if I had come from a more established background (established in terms of upper crust society), I would have developed more options during my post-secondary education. Yet I never realized how pinned in I had become until I began to look outside Medicine.

I had become a primary care physician. I was a revenue generator. In the eyes of my employer, I had an expected productivity and associated costs. I had to cover my costs in order to make myself valuable to my organization. Based on current compensation rates for seeing people in an office setting, my productivity demands precluded me from having adequate time to address all, or even most of the issues of concern to my patients. I tried to be understanding and cover as much as possible. I knew they had to wait at least 3 months to get an appointment to see me again. As a result, I was always running late. Well, how could I stay on time when I only had 20 minutes to talk to a patient who might well pull out a list of 5 questions from their pocket when I entered the room. I knew I was fortunate to have 20 minute appointments versus the 10 minutes I often heard about in news stories (but didn't know if they actually existed). However, it generally took me 30 minutes to cover a patient's issues in sufficient detail, so we both left with a better understanding of what needed to happen to manage their medical problems effectively.

Was it too much to ask for this kind of time to talk to my patients? My boss seemed to think so. I could ask for less money, for changes in my schedule, for whatever else I wanted, but the bottom line always seemed to be the same, productivity. I was required to see more patients, as revenues never seemed to meet the institution's expectations.

What was wrong with our health care system? Health Maintenance Organizations (HMOs) often took the rap. The high cost of drugs was another target. Surely, some of this was deserved. Yet I felt the problems in health care extended well beyond their borders. I believed it was time that we, the doctors, started shouldering more of the blame. We were the ones who saw the patients, and if we ultimately took a stand that it was important to be able to sit down and talk to people so that we could better understand their issues, we could make it happen.

In January of 2000, a colleague of mine, who was usually incredibly busy with his part time clinical practice, saw a couple of my patients for urgent visits (related to upper respiratory infections). When I noted he had seen them, I sent him an e-mail thanking him. He said it was not a problem, as a new patient had canceled, so it was easy to fit them in to his schedule. He noted his 4 hour session that day was quite pleasant, as he had only 9 patients to see, and felt like he was able to attend to all the issues presented, without feeling harried, or in need of cutting a patient short.

I felt such a statement was pathetic. Why couldn't most days be like that? Why did that have to be the exception and not the rule? I often told patients, "You don't like the way my schedule is set up, as it's hard to get in to see me, and I'm always running late. I surely don't like it as I feel incredible pressure to stay on time, so who benefits from it?". I have explored some of the factors and entities which have contributed to the current practice of health care, and what we might be able to do to fix it. We need to permit health care to devolve back into a system where patients, and their issues are the primary consideration, and not a secondary issue, addressed only in slick marketing material.

Chapter 2

"Doc"

Somewhere between the eighth and ninth grades I transitioned from wanting to be a dentist to a doctor. Of course, there was no clear, rational basis for this decision. Why I was ever interested in dentistry was also unclear to me. I had no role models, nor any particular interest in teeth (I didn't even like brushing my teeth, and hadn't even heard of flossing at that time). However, at the time I was drawn to a Reader's Digest series "I am Joe's….(body part)". As a 12 year old, I found this fascinating. I would excitedly wait for my next issue of Reader's Digest to arrive, so I could read the next installment of "Joe's body".

My interest in Medicine continued into high school despite my grades not being particularly good. It never seemed very important to me that they be good, but of course, I had no way of knowing if grades truly were important. I went to a high school where only 10% of the graduates went on to college, many attending a community college. Thus, striving for good grades didn't seem to be particularly valuable. Despite my average grades through the first part of my junior year in high school, my friends and family weren't deterred from calling me "Doc". At some level, they felt that I would ultimately succeed in this endeavor (my parents seemed to have more doubts about my success than others I knew). Finally, halfway through my junior year, my relationship with Matt, a friend who was an intellectual equal, and who was also interested in Medicine (largely because his Dad was the only doctor in town), sparked a new interest in academics. As my math teacher recalled at our Senior Awards Dinner, I got "turned on" (which of course, had many meanings in those days). My math turn on occurred when we studied trigonometry in the eleventh grade. Trigonometry proved sufficiently difficult to make it unintelligible to people who worked hard, but didn't have great analytical skills. I was finally at an advantage. I had excellent analytical skills and the ability to understand abstract information and concepts. Yet still, I was lacking in any kind of study habits. If I couldn't finish my homework before class was over, and stick it in my school book, it usually didn't get done.

That wasn't totally true my senior year, when I took Advance Placement English. Being a slow reader, I was forced to read at home so I could talk intelligently about the literature in class. When I had taken my SATs, I was quite deficient in language skills (480) but above average in math (720). Overall, this was more than enough to get into the University of Michigan (UM), the only college to which I applied. It was ironic that despite the limitations of my public high school and my poor SAT score in language skills, I was able to place out of not only first year calculus, but also freshman English.

My first glimpse of applying for medical school came when I filled out my application for UM. I noticed that they had a program called Inteflex. This was a combined undergraduate/medical school program that had a student on the hospital wards in 4 years (instead of the more typical six or more years). Of course, I had no idea that I really needed to have been on the ball in high school to get into such a program, but at the time, it was easy enough to check off the box. UM decided I didn't quite cut it for the Inteflex program, but they did offer me a place in LS&A (the college of Literature, Science and Arts).

I found my entrance into college quite liberating. I was finally in an environment where brains and thought were valued (as opposed to hair style and music preference). In addition, there was such a wide range of topics to pursue. I delved into the usual pre-medical studies, but also started taking classes outside of science, such as philosophy and German.

My science training in high school was rather limited, so being able to take a slew of science courses was quite exciting. I was especially looking forward to biochemistry. In fact, the dreaded organic chemistry turned out to be a breeze. Just as in trigonometry in high school, it was one of those topics that required abstract thinking skills. I never got a 100% on an organic test, but because they graded to the mean, I was able to get an "A+". In fact, the only "B" I got in a college science class was a "B+" in my freshman chemistry lab.

My failure to get an "A" in chemistry lab was an insightful experience. I was becoming familiar with the scientific concept that we should faithfully and honestly record the experimental data we generated. Unfortunately, the calorimeter experiment we performed required us to use rather limited materials: a Styrofoam® cup filled with water which was covered with tin foil and had a thermometer in the center. Our task was to measure the heat capacity of water (this result was well known to us as 1 calorie per cubic centimeter). The calorimeter I made was so inaccurate that I completely failed the experiment. The numbers I generated were in marked conflict to the known heat capacity of water, and thus, I had built a defective calorimeter. My faulty data became the entire focus of the experiment. The fact that I understood the concept of heat capacity and the conceptual aspects of its measurement were irrelevant to the teaching assistant. I could have easily fudged the data, knowing the desired result before the experiment even began. Yet, my faithful recording of the experimental data became my downfall. So much for rewarding honesty!

The "B+" wasn't a major blow, however. I had enough "A"s to end up with a 3.8 grade point average, substantially better than my 3.1 grade point average from high school. Some of my friends in college also called me "Doc", as they heard my high school friends use the term when they visited. Again, I wasn't particularly worried about getting into medical (med) school. I had read the college bulletin on the first day of school, and knew exactly what courses to take (i.e. requirements for admission to med school). I lined up my letters of recommendation as I went along, and gained some hospital experience via my uncle's connections at a Detroit area hospital. I thought I was rounding out my experiences as expected, only to find out I really didn't have a clue.

Just as with college, the only med school I wanted to go to was UM's. Why ever leave Ann Arbor if you didn't have to, I thought? I applied for their early decision program, which required me to apply to only a single med school. In turn I would be notified by September 1st if I was accepted or not. Figuring my acceptance was perfunctory, I entered the early decision process. My confidence about getting into UM faded the morning I met a hard nosed physician during my first interview.

I had set up my med school interview for 8am on a Friday. That summer I was working at Hydramatic, a large General Motors factory in neighboring Ypsilanti, Michigan. I worked midnights, so generally I would get home around 7am. That fateful Friday after I returned from work, I showered, ate a big breakfast, and laid out my suit before lying on the couch for a little pre-interview rest. I awoke staring at the large clock in front of me. It was 8am, the time my interview down the street was supposed to begin. Since I had to get a move on, I threw on my clothes, and headed to the nearby med school. It was raining, but I made it in the door with umbrella in hand at 8:15 am. Just as I walked to the desk to sign in, a physician came out and said, "I guess this Sobieraj (mispronounced, of course) guy isn't coming".

I assured him that indeed I had come, and apologized for my tardiness. At that point I found out that Medicine was potentially stuffier than I could ever have imagined. He asked me if I knew what an HMO was. Though this question is easily answered today, it was not so easy in August of 1979. He told me it was the future of Medicine (he was unfortunately correct on that point). He proceeded to ask me about my interest in culture. For example, had I ever been to the Detroit Institute of Arts? I assured him I hadn't. He told me that I was much too science oriented, and should have broadened my background.

I left there with the writing on the wall that I would be leaving Ann Arbor by the fall of 1980. It finally became clear to me why pre-meds (students trying to get into medical school) I knew when I first arrived at UM spent so much time taking introductory psychology courses. They wanted to be (appear) well-rounded. People from backgrounds which taught them how to play the med school entry game had a path clearly outlined for them. They knew which classes and activities gave "the look" on their applications. All I ever did was study what interested and excited me.

I realized that people from working class backgrounds, without a prior link to Medicine, had a real struggle against such narrow minded physician interviewers. Why didn't it matter that I had been to Tiger Stadium or the Olympia a million times (where the Detroit Tigers and Red Wings played, respectively)? I could have given him detailed stories about events there. Why didn't he ask me how it was working in auto factories in the summer so I could pay for my schooling? I could have told him about the putrid air I had to breathe everyday and how I had come to realize why so many people smoked in that environment. None of that seemed to matter.

Fortunately, my interview at Wayne State University in Detroit went substantially better. The interviewer did comment on my poor writing skills; evidently not much improved since my SAT days. However, despite this deficiency, they let me in. I was finally able to begin MY medical career.

Chapter 3

Wayne's World

My wife feels it was prophetic that I went to Wayne State University (Wayne). We met on the first day of school, as the alphabet found us in close proximity. I had decided that the first week of med school was going to be largely review, so I had planned to go back-packing on the Bruce Peninsula in Canada instead. She was sufficiently impressed by my disregard for being anxious about starting med school that we hit it off. However, the fact that our first date was to watch the horror of the Reagan landslide over Jimmy Carter, wasn't a great way to start. Yet we made it through together, and without her, I wouldn't have spent the past 17 years in Boston, which has been a good experience overall (as a patient of mine once said, "Detroit is a good place to be from").

Medical students tend to segregate themselves early into their destined specialties. I was always an abstract thinker. Thus, I found biochemistry, immunology and physiology interesting. Anatomy was boring, something to be tolerated as we learned where things were in the body. This made me destined for internal medicine. What about the people (largely guys) who liked anatomy? They became surgeons. If they were jocks in addition to liking anatomy, orthopedic surgery (especially if they liked to crack jokes during physiology seminars).

My attraction to Medicine was inevitable. I suspect I would have done some minor things differently if I had to do it over again. Yet even today, I suspect my interests would have drawn me to math and science, again. Over time the math and science would have became overly technical as I moved into advanced courses. At that point, I would need the biologic aspect of my studies to sustain me, once again. Since I liked working with people, and didn't like the idea of being stuck behind a laboratory bench top mixing solutions, I was destined to be a clinician. It seems it would have been hard to alter that pathway, even today.

In reality, my background was quite diverse, which ultimately was an asset when I became a primary care physician. My working class background made familiarity with the views and habits of working people second nature. The summers spent working in auto factories enabled close contact with a breadth of ethnic diversity. Also, my experience at UM gave me the background for dealing with educated people. In fact, my medical training had best prepared me for dealing with educated people. However, it was having facility with uneducated people, or people of simple means and understanding, that was never taught. My background gave me comfort in this regard, allowing me to communicate instinctively with less educated people.

Another thing we learned in med school was how to deal with the medical system. As in all professions, there was an order to this system. The paths that people took through the medical system could be defined, learned, and when appropriate, repeated. We learned how to structure our days so that we could have our clinical interactions mixed in with other activities. In med school, the non-patient care activities were educational sessions referred to as didactics. The didactics could involve attending a class or lecture, or simply reading clinically related material. Later, when actually practicing Medicine, the other activities would include some administration/paper work (often onerous), and/or research/teaching.

The evolution of a medical student into a resident (a.k.a. house officer) was a truly laissez-faire process. There was essentially no pressure dictating what field one went into. Despite this, as I alluded to above, there was a tendency for an unconscious matching of personality type to specialty. One of the advantages of going to a state school like Wayne was the large class size. In fact, the 256 students in our class was the largest of any in the country, but typical for Wayne. Thus, a broad range of personality types were represented. Some of the more socially inept aptly chose non-patient care fields such as pathology or radiology. This was good, as it would have been frightening to think that some of my classmates would actually be taking care of people.

We were taught in med school to listen to people. We were taught how to ask questions, both to get useful, unbiased information, and to obtain it in a sensitive manner. We truly could learn these skills, even if we came to med school without them. The characteristics we were required to bring with us to med school included a sense of caring, responsibility and patience. In many ways, time didn't matter. What else would we be doing anyway, playing softball? Few of us were married, and fewer still had kids. So we could begin to devote ourselves to our careers.

Unfortunately, as we became more integrated into the clinical realm, we learned other less desirable behaviors. We learned that when you are running out of time, you ask a short, specific question, and hear only what you think is important in the response. We learned how to get patients through the system, as though we had created the system ourselves. Some of these skills would be necessary for survival, and others would become practical aids, a part of our profession.

We began seeing real patients during our third year of med school. These were people who were sick or seeing their doctor for a specific reason as opposed to the people who were paid to act as patients during our earliest clinical exercises in the first and second years of med school. During these early visits with real patients, we were given ample time to accomplish our goals. We learned how to take a history and perform a physical. We learned all the questions necessary to fully evaluate a system of the body, such as the cardiovascular system. We learned specific procedural skills (e.g. drawing blood) and physical exam maneuvers (e.g. how to detect ascites, which is fluid in the abdomen). As we progressed through our training, we had less and less time to see each patient. This was the beginning of the process of efficiency. The underlying, and I believe, still untested assumption in medical training which posited that by gaining experience, we would become more efficient (and thus, faster).

Indeed, I am sure we became more efficient. In part, this was because we learned what not to ask, as well as which questions to ask. This saved time, as we gave the patient fewer questions to answer. In addition, theoretically we arrive at a diagnosis more quickly, and perform a physical exam more ably. However, an alternative hypothesis would be that an experienced physician would take even longer per visit over time. The experienced clinician would see nuances the youngster missed, and thus, would be compelled to follow up on them. In addition, the experienced clinician would have a greater wealth of information to share with patients about their particular issues, due to the physician's greater breadth of knowledge. Today I could tell a patient much more about a high cholesterol level than I could have 15 years ago. This was in part, because I knew more about what it meant in a practical sense, but also because I had seen 15 years' worth of data played out in front of me, building on the historical mound of information I accrued as a medical student.

In summary, the not-so-subtle, real life lessons we learned at Wayne were just as important and equally assimilated as the specific knowledge our instructors taught us. They said their goal was for us to become caring, dedicated physicians. Yet the system they introduced us to began to erode those precepts before we even graduated. From there, it was just a matter of time before we learned the way things really worked in Medicine. We could no longer avoid the underlying forces that drove the health care system we had entered. We would become masters at processing patients.

Chapter 4

Beantown

My wife and I proceeded through the interview phase for residency as we planned our choices for the upcoming Residency Match ("the Match" is a national process that connects med school graduates with post-doctoral training programs (known as residencies) in such fields as medicine, surgery, obstetrics, etc.). During the interviewing season, I climbed into my suit, and tried to make myself sound impressive. I had the grades and honor societies behind me, and as a result I wanted to go to a good program. I fell in love with Seattle when I was out there in October of 1983, but my wife, who was going to become a psychiatrist, found their psychiatry program antithetical to the type of psychiatry she was interested in. We had to go to a city acceptable to both of us, which had attractive programs in both internal medicine and psychiatry. Since we were both Yankees, we narrowed the choice to Chicago and Boston. Boston was our first choice, as it was smaller and more manageable than Chicago, in addition to having very good programs in both fields. We had a match list of over 50 permutations of our respective choices. In retrospect, it seemed a waste of time, as I got into my first Boston choice, and my wife her second.

The energy and enthusiasm generated by my internship (the first year of residency) was remarkable. It was a culmination of the educational process. I had learned a lot, and now it was time to apply it. An intern becomes the responsible person for all his/her patients. In reality, there was also a supervising resident and an attending (supervising) physician, but we, the interns, felt and were made to feel by others that we were the "man".

Internship was also draining due to its persistent demands. In our post-graduate training we experienced an even more profound indoctrination into the medical system. The medical training establishment allowed residents to buck the system to some extent, but social pressure toward greater conformity became important. It was not that one couldn't continue to function in an eclectic and possibly rebellious fashion, but that there were certain "rules" about how the system worked. While these were not formal rules, many of the unwritten ones were tacitly endorsed by the top of the pyramid, and were perceived to be validated by the public at large. This might be best understood by an example.

The hallowed white coat was clearly a revered symbol. This was reinforced at Boston University (BU) by the White Coat Ceremony. During a formal introduction ceremony, third year medical students entering their clinical clerkships would don a white coat for the first time. This was problematic in many senses. One problem related to a concept developed by the German philosopher Fuerbach, and used by Karl Marx in his protest of capitalism. That was the concept of alienation. Alienation refers to the distancing one has from an object or belief when a part of the internal human spirit is projected outside one's self. The concept of alienation may be better understood by considering the case of God. As Fuerbach would posit, by taking who we are as humans, perfecting it in an ideal form, and calling it God, we create a distance between ourselves, the actual human, and this perfected abstraction of our human selves. The perfected abstraction, God, when it is projected outside of ourselves into an external entity, comes to gain power it doesn't have before this externalization of the ideal human. As a consequence of this external projection of ourselves, we become alienated from the internal human qualities we have projected as God. These qualities are no longer seen as a part of us, but of this idealized, external agent. Physicians have done this with the white coat, giving it greater meaning and value than it has deserved, and in turn, a power the white coat could never have mustered on its own.

The white coat of a doctor had become an externalization of who the doctor really was inside the coat. The white coat had become a symbol of what took place in a person when training to be a doctor. This imagery was quite powerful. In fact, it was so strong that it even had a disorder named after it. "White coat hypertension" referred to people whose blood pressures were normal in their everyday lives, but would increase when they saw their doctor. I had joked with patients, that they couldn't have white coat hypertension with me, since I didn't wear one. Yet the reality was, I did have several patients who had manifested this phenomenon (which was easily documented by a 24 hour blood pressure monitor).

Thus, the white coat had become quite an important symbol of who we were as doctors. Over the years, many weight loss clinics have enhanced their image by dressing all their non-MD staff in white coats for their ads. In fact, the symbol was so important that at my hospital a couple of years ago, the Vice Chair of Clinical Affairs in the Department of Medicine wrote in a memo that all doctors needed to wear white coats in the hospital and clinic or wear their hospital IDs, so that people could tell who the doctors were. He even noted that the first choice of identification would be a white coat, and the hospital ID second.

As a result, I started brandishing my ID about my neck. Two years after this edict, many non-MDs in the hospital continued to wear white coats, including dietitians, nurse case managers, ward clerks, etc. So it seems we ultimately ended up with hospital IDs for distinguishing physicians from the rest of the crowd (if indeed such a distinction was necessary).

My second favorite MD symbol was the tie. Being male, I had been dealt the tie hand. I decided in my third year of med school that a tie wasn't for me. Recognizing the conformity issues present back then, I realized I couldn't always get away without one, so I would occasionally wear a tie. However, in due time, I concluded there weren't real barriers to not wearing a tie, only the ones I had fabricated in my own mind.

Now this wasn't totally true. When I saw patients, I had no problem convincing them that I was indeed a physician. By my manner, the questions I asked, the answers I gave, and the exams I did, patients had no problem discerning in their first encounter with me that, indeed, I was a physician. So, it didn't appear that the barrier to accepting a tieless physician was on the patients' side. The attitudinal barrier was really at the higher end of the medical pyramid. I had learned that those at the top really did have a concept of how an MD should appear. They would also in some cases, hold it against one if he or she didn't have a particular look. By "hold it against", I mean that every time a staff physician was picked for an assignment or task, the presence or lack of a tie and/or white coat became a factor that was considered in the decision. Race may not be allowed to be a consideration in such decisions, but white coats and ties were acceptable criteria to help guide decisions. After all, there was an image that needed to be conveyed.

In general, I had taken the view that I would just let my actions speak for me. This had worked well for the most part, and had allowed me to achieve at a high level. Yet I knew my style had been a barrier to advancement at times, and thus, something that I had to learn to accept. I suspect at times, not getting a position, or being pulled from one where I had literally been told I was doing a good job had more to do with my casual style than substance.

What was OK for a resident (in terms of dress and style) was not necessarily the case for attending physicians (those of us at a more established level who supervised the training of interns, residents and fellows). The assumption was that all trainees should outgrow such tendencies, and those that didn't, may have had a lesion (i.e. defect) somewhere which should be carefully monitored. So, in addition, to learning a lot of Medicine, and how to manage critically ill patients, I became imbued with the Medicine etiquette. Unfortunately, I came to the conclusion that I didn't like this etiquette. In fact, I had hoped that they (the medical establishment) would get over it, and stop holding it against me as opposed to my eventually conceding to the white coat, tie, etc.

The other point I should make about style was that it was also specialty dependent. For example, there were two large groups of MDs in the operating room (OR), the surgeons and the anesthesiologists. They two groups appeared identical in the OR. Both sets of doctors wore surgical "scrubs".

Yet, before going into the OR, or while in the hospital at large, their appearances couldn't have been more different. The anesthesiologists came in dressed in relatively casual clothing, sometimes downright laid back. They may have worn ties, but definitely not a suit and only occasionally a sport coat.

On the other hand, surgeons, it seemed, could spend an hour getting ready in the morning, put on a three piece suit, come into the hospital, go directly to the OR, and take it all off only to put on scrubs. They would then re-dress after their OR cases, so they could look sharp once again. The white coat, when worn by a surgeon, would be perfectly buttoned up. Flowing tails from an unbuttoned white coat was definitely not acceptable (even amongst Surgical House Staff). If a surgeon didn't wear a white coat, a suit appeared to be mandatory, not optional.

If you think I am kidding, take a look at the apparel of the different MDs you come into contact with in the next 5 years. You will be able to guess their specialty 90% of the time based solely on their dress (this is my conjecture; I have no specific data supporting this statement).

As you can see, medical training was quite robust. It not only helped us to understand better the science on which Medicine was based, it also helped us to become familiar with the medical system. We learned how to process patients efficiently (and how to become indignant when this didn't happen). We learned how the class system in Medicine worked, and the need for conformity in this non-codified system. Finally, we were left with enough skill and ideas that we could go out into the real world, and try to fix all that we had identified as being wrong with the medical system.

Chapter 5

Hanging out a Shingle

There was such a social component to becoming a physician. As I proceeded through my training, people would ask me when I was going to "hang out my shingle". They seemed to long for the days when health care appeared to be simpler. Hanging out one's shingle was a way of introducing oneself to a community, and thus, becoming a member of it. During my training, most of my fellow residents weren't sure they were ready to hang out their shingles. Many were looking at fellowships to train as subspecialists (e.g. cardiologists), while others were looking at General Practice opportunities. Most practice opportunities meant joining a group, and assimilating into the culture of the particular practice.

A practice's culture could be quite varied. Some groups had an academic focus (rare), while most focused on productivity and efficiency. Productivity looked at how one's billing practices compared to others', and efficiency pertained to how low one could keep their overhead. It seemed to me, that as one became acclimated to primary care as part of a group practice, they would assimilate into the business world. It was often stated in med school that one needed a business degree to practice Medicine. While this may have seemed to be the case to our largely business ignorant profession, the business skills actually required to run a practice were few and well defined.

Since I never fit the mold of such a group practice, in 1990, I set out to build a private, solo practice. This of course was not a common mode for starting a practice at the time. Most physicians at the hospitals to which I admitted patients were members of a group. However, there were a few of us who practiced solo. After discussing the nuances of this process with my solo colleagues, I believed I could gradually grow such a practice.

I was fortunate at the time, to have been involved with a weight loss program at the hospital where I served as Chief Medical Resident. My predecessor as Medical Director of the program had ambitions of striking it big in corporate medicine, and had hoped to move on. Since he and I were of similar academic ilk, I was his logical successor when he finally did move on to Sandoz Nutrition's corporate offices in Minneapolis in 1990.

I became director of the largest OptiFast® Program in New England. This might have been quite a statement in the late 1980s. But as Oprah regained her weight, the OptiFast® veneer began to lose its luster. I remained fully committed to the idea that people could ultimately improve their nutrition, and thus, their quality of life. Yet, OptiFast® gave the impression of a fad diet (as explicitly stated by my wife one day, much to my annoyance).

In April of 1990, I founded "Preventive and Nutritional Medicine". I had gained some marketing experience via the OptiFast® Program, and felt I wanted my corporate name to reflect my belief system. I believed in the premise, if you build it, they will come. However, I soon learned that no matter how good I was as a physician, and no matter how good my ideas may have been, it wasn't easy to get people to change their patterns of behavior. In addition, efforts to function as a nutrition specialist were not supported by referrals from colleagues. Their concerns ranged from fears of losing patients to me, to frank ignorance of what was appropriate nutrition for patients with particular medical issues.

I had always been amazed that even the most academic of physicians derived most of their knowledge about nutrition from sources like Jane Brody at the New York Times. In the days of evidence based medicine, when we were supposed to use only practices that were supported by randomized, controlled clinical trials, our views about nutrition had been formed earlier in our lives. Many of the foolish things we learned in grade school would be profoundly reiterated to our patients as fact. Somehow silly ideas, when spoken authoritatively by someone wearing a white coat, became more valid. A common fallacy was the primacy of breakfast as the most important meal of the day. My attempts to find data to support this statement over the years were fruitless. I came to the conclusion that this concept was likely a marketing strategy created by the cereal industry (Dr. Kellogg in the early part of the twentieth century spent much time trying to make breakfast a nutritious fare, something health food stores would be proud of today, but quite unlike what his name brand cereal company sells as "nutritious" in the year 2000).

Using sound nutritional advice, along with other lifestyle changes, and prudent internal medicine, I hoped to provide outstanding primary care. I also had the good fortune of being able to connect with people. Whether they were indigent, blue collar, or business class, I could speak to them in their language. I always tried to stress a lifestyle change before trying medication, especially when there was no short term danger associated with a patient's condition.

Since a growing practice has holes in the schedule, it was easy to spend sufficient time with my patients initially. However, as I got busy, it became more difficult. Yet, being my own boss enabled me to ensure that my schedule wasn't overly crowded. This permitted me to be both on time, and also to have adequate time to address the issues people brought to their visits with me. In private, solo practice, I was able to practice a simple business dictum. Profitability could be driven by a high throughput with little efficiency, or by having a lower throughput, but with improved efficiency. Both could maintain a positive bottom line, and I chose the latter business model.

Most practitioners I encountered had high throughputs with little efficiency (similar to my current practice at an academic medical center). Patients were squeezed in at any possible moment, with little concern as to what they were coming in for, what their needs might be, and whether their needs would be adequately met in the time allotted. Due to the overwhelming demands of third party billing rules and requirements, most practices had plentiful office staff. There were people to check in patients, others to assist the physician in getting people ready, or to perform tests, if needed. Finally others would manage referrals, and other paperwork related to billing, etc. Most practices would estimate that their overhead ran at 40-50%.

Such a low efficiency was particularly unappealing to me, as I saw it as a requirement to see many more patients per hour than I desired. I had a goal of 20% overhead. Most of the 20% would be my secretary and rent for my office space. However, this meant that many clinical responsibilities fell on my shoulders. My secretary was experienced working in medical offices, and could adequately triage calls (i.e. decide who needed to be called back first). Yet, I did all weights, blood pressures, vaccinations, ECGs (electrocardiograms), blood draws, etc., things that non-MD staff do in traditional practices. Much of this was not inappropriate as the rationale for not having physicians do it in busy practices has to do with productivity (i.e. physicians having as many visits that pay as much as possible in the time they are there). Anything that distracted from that, whether helpful to the patient or not, was shunned in most practices.

I was able to meet my overhead goal, and thus, support my salary needs before I left private practice (modest salary needs, indeed, by current standards in primary care). I had even interviewed a woman who I thought would have been a good partner in growing the practice further before I left. Well, if things were so good, why did I leave the confines and control of a private solo practice for a chaotic, group practice in the city?

There were several factors. Some of them related to petty politics while others had to do with the amount of time I had to spend billing insurance companies and processing referrals to other providers in order to keep my overhead down. I had excellent practice software for managing these issues, but despite this, it was still quite onerous. This was in part due to the many billing and referral rules each insurer had, and also by the continual need to update my practice software to accommodate all billing changes issued by insurers. However, for me the straw that broke the camel's back was capitation.

Capitation was derived from the term per capita (literally Latin for per body). I had refused to become a provider for the insurance company US health care because they had a capitated program. They would have paid me $100 a year to take care of a healthy young woman. Unfortunately, that would only cover her annual physical and PAP smear. If she had any lifestyle issues which needed modification or any other medical needs, it would be at my expense. This type of capitated system was viewed as acceptable by colleagues of mine who practiced conventional internal medicine. That was, out of sight, out of mind. If the patient didn't complain about something, they assumed it wasn't broken. Colleagues of mine told me how great it was that a significant subset of their patients wouldn't even come in for visits. Thus, for those patients, they were paid the capitation fee for having these patients list them as their primary care provider without having to provide them any service at all.

With the type of Medicine I was practicing, this couldn't work. I would feel it was incumbent on me to make sure they had annual exams. If they were overweight, had a tendency toward diabetes, smoked, or were physically inactive, I would be compelled to see them a few times a year, if not more often, to try and improve their habits. Thus, I couldn't accept a system such as US Healthcare's. The problem was, that in the mid-1990s, there was talk of many other insurers moving to a capitated system of payment. Thus, I feared I wouldn't be able to avoid the capitation juggernaut.

I felt compelled to look for a group to join, so I could share the risk of sick patients who might drain my budget. I also felt that moving to a supportive, like minded group would allow me to continue to practice with a nutritional and preventive focus. My return to the institution where I did my residency seemed to fit the bill, though I ultimately came to learn, I couldn't have been more wrong.

Chapter 6

Welcome to
Corporate Medicine!

As it turned out, I had gone from one extreme to another. In private practice I was all alone as a clinician, and in total control of my immediate environment. In the group I joined, I was surrounded by other clinicians, and had marginal control of my environment. What I desired to control most was my schedule. This was what gave me the time to see my patients, and meet their needs. When I was interviewing for jobs, I made sure that the appointments were scheduled a minimum of 20 minutes for a return visit. In addition, in my new practice, new patients were given 50 minute visits, which was generally adequate to cover most issues (if not all, depending on the complexity of a patient's past medical history).

What I didn't realize until after my arrival, was that double booking (i.e. scheduling a second person at the same time as a currently scheduled patient) was not only accepted but encouraged. The clerical staff often had little regard for how tightly booked a schedule was, nor its impact on the patients and the clinicians who cared for them. For example, a clinical session (a block of clinic time in which patients are scheduled for appointments) that began with two patients in the first twenty minute slot (i.e. double booking), in my experience, inevitably led all subsequent visits that session to be late. Double booking exacerbated the basic tendency my patient had of having more issues to address than could be managed in a twenty minute session. As a result, I would end up running further and further behind in my schedule.

In addition, my boss and I had quite different practice styles. He practiced conventional medicine, which often paid little attention to lifestyle and nutrition. His approach to nutrition was to refer patients to a dietitian. In some cases this was clearly necessary to allow patients adequate time to ask detailed questions and develop an appropriate meal plan. However, when a diabetic patient came for a return visit with poor glucose control, the issue wasn't just whether he or she needed more diabetic medication. Just as a business could have higher profits by operating more efficiently, diabetics could have better blood sugar control by putting less stress on their insulin system (the hormone system which regulates blood sugar). When one actually added this nutritional approach to the management of a patient's medications, you may readily see why this approach couldn't be accomplished in twenty minutes. As a way of getting around the time dilemma, a senior colleague in my General Medicine Section recommended that I stretch out the discussion of a particular diet over 4-5 patient visits. Unfortunately, such an ignorant comment underlined one of the difficulties of bringing nutrition into a primary care practice. Often patients had to replace a food in their diet with another, more healthful food, or more likely, several foods would need to be modified at once. In addition, good nutritional practice required one to identify high risk foods which patients needed to modify first, with secondary modifications based on how well they responded to the initial change. Each aspect of the meal plan needed to be viewed as a unit, that worked together. This was in contrast to the narrowly acting medications we used in our conventional practice of Medicine.

This ultimately led to the view amongst my superiors that my running late, and spending 30 minutes with a patient was volitional, and due to my inefficiencies. The fact that patients may actually be getting broader care wasn't considered a possibility. The logic was if one physician could work a session in the allotted time, then all clinical sessions would be held to the same time constraints. Patient care was not considered to suffer by such time constraints. Of course, I hadn't shown in a randomized, controlled trial that my way was better. Thus, this argument on my part wasn't considered tenable. Yet time constraints were only one of many issues I had with corporate medicine.

Health insurance (i.e. third party) reimbursement actually favored corporate medicine over a simpler, smaller focus of care. It was analogous to cheese made by Kraft versus that made by a dairy farmer in Vermont. The latter could make a fine, economically viable product, as well as the former, except when we stacked the deck against them (e.g. corporate subsidies and tax breaks that actually gave a commercial edge to the large company). Well such an edge was also given to corporate medicine. In addition, corporate medicine included hospitals, free standing clinics and other patient care entities where generating revenue was the primary concern.

Of course all clinical entities need to generate revenue or they will cease to exist. I generated plenty of revenue in my private practice. At times while in practice, I even became corrupted by the billing process. For example, if I saw a patient and spent 1/2 an hour with them discussing and evaluating their medical problems, I could bill a 99214 (a number, or billing code, used to refer to a level of service provided to an established patient). However, I could generate even more revenue by giving a cortisone shot in someone's elbow for tendonitis. So when I saw someone with tendonitis, I could and did bill the more expensive procedure to maximize my revenue. This was actually legal. However, a problem existed when marginally necessary tests and procedures were done largely to generate revenue. Some physicians would perform an ECG on all patients over 40 who were seen for an annual physical. While this might make sense from a patient's perspective, to a physician, it makes no clinical sense. A routine ECG was of little to no predictive value in a person without symptoms referable to the heart, if they were also at low risk for developing heart disease. Yet, it was a great way to add $45-50 of revenue to the coffers that day.

This is a minor example, but exemplifies a common problem in clinical situations where the provider of the service directly benefits financially from the service provided. I have told patients that if they were interested in a surgical opinion, and were not really sure they wanted to go through with the procedure, go to a surgeon who was very busy. I believed they were less likely to pursue unnecessary surgery, as their schedule was already overburdened, and didn't need to include unnecessary operations.

Some medical procedures could have quite varied indications (i.e. reasons for doing them), and thus, the provider had a lot of latitude in deciding if a test or procedure was necessary. One such procedure was cardiac catheterization (also called a "cath" or "cardiac cath"). This procedure generated approximately $10,000 each time it was done. Many hospitals have gone to great efforts to establish cardiac catheterization laboratories for this reason. (In fact, Christmas week 2000, the local National Public Radio station carried a news report that three community hospitals were going to get Massachusetts' approval to do coronary bypass surgery, with revenue enhancement one of the primary objectives). However, with respect to heart disease, attempts at maximizing medical therapy and lifestyle modification were often circumvented by the easier path of offering the patient the quick fix via the catheter. A patient could take a particular medication for the rest of their life, give up many foods they were eating, and start exercising to prevent their coronary artery disease from progressing, or a cardiologist could take the same patient into the cath lab, put a balloon into the blockage and *voila*, the patient would be all set. Of course, the patient might still need to deal with that lifestyle stuff, but they potentially could do that later (which often meant never). By August of 1999, there was finally sound data (B Pitt, et al, New England Journal of Medicine) which showed that the approach of medication, diet and exercise was actually superior to the cardiac catheterization approach. Has this discouraged catheterizations? If it has, I doubt nearly enough. An extreme approach would be to compensate cardiac caths by paying $1000 for the procedure. This level of compensation wouldn't cover the costs of doing the procedure, but it would surely eliminate unnecessary caths.

Yet what has really favored corporate medicine over the small guy (e.g. a solo practitioner) is facility fees. A facility fee is paid to hospitals and clinics over and above what is paid for the actual procedure (here I use the term to mean a service of any kind). Thus, when I saw a patient in my private office for which I paid rent, I was reimbursed X dollars. Now when I saw the same patient at my hospital's clinic, the hospital was paid 2X on my behalf. They received the same fee that I received when in private practice, plus an additional fee of equal amount to the service fee paid, to cover the costs of maintaining the facility. This fee was something that had been negotiated by hospitals in the 1970s, and with the financial squeeze that had been placed on reimbursement for routine care, had made it almost impossible to have a small efficient practice, as I once had.

The corporate medical center was not only corrupted by the development of revenue enhancing procedures. They also effectively eliminated services which were not generating adequate revenue. In the fall of 2000, my local, community newspaper carried several stories about strategic planning cuts at community hospitals. This translated into the following: when a service (e.g. obstetrics) becomes a revenue loser, the hospital would eliminate the service and stem the tide. Consideration of offering a smaller service more efficiently (e.g. a birthing center that encompassed part of a ward instead of all 20-30 beds) wasn't an option. There wasn't time for such redesign issues. Hospitals needed to make the cuts, and move on. Revenue generation was the primary focus.

Both of the two communities served by my local paper had community hospitals. The larger hospital of the two had grown their birthing center enormously in the 1990s, with more than 3000 live births annually (and believe me, they'd like to see 4000). On the other hand, the smaller hospital attempted to save their obstetrics unit (or birthing center). They needed less than 1000 (about 800) live births to have that center pay for itself. However, under the design they chose, they could never meet this goal, and the strategic planning move was to lop it off (i.e. close it).

Ultimately, from a public policy perspective, shifting all obstetric care to one hospital could result in an efficient regional use of hospitals. All the births from the two communities could be performed in a single hospital. The problem from my perspective was more the style that a corporate mentality brought. First and foremost was the bottom line, and all hospital departments had to attend to this. In order for a negative bottom line to be tolerated by a department, it had to be a critical service (e.g. an Emergency Room). If not, it was expendable. Yet the marketing and competitive forces present made a rational change nearly impossible. The marketing people at the smaller community hospital above wanted to keep as positive an image as possible for their birthing center. Despite the red ink, they tried to keep up appearances, in order to maintain their current customers. When they decided to eliminate the service, there was little to no warning. Their obstetrics unit went from being a great place to have a baby (marketing) to one that couldn't make it (competitive). These two elements functioned together in an antagonistic way which prevented rational planning. There was no time to develop creative solutions, as the corporate bottom line (profit) had to be adhered to.

Another offshoot of corporate medicine has been the specialty hospital. Specialty hospitals are not a new phenomenon. New England Baptist Hospital has long been known for its orthopedic surgery, and little else. I was never sure if they even offered primary care services. Corporate medicine encouraged this hospital (known locally as "the Baptist") to pick off one of the most lucrative services in Medicine, joint replacements (e.g. a hip or knee replacement).

At times, in order to increase revenues, corporate planning encourages a hospital to enter a new market, such as substance abuse. The hospital tries to obtain insurance contracts, which would require people with that insurance to go to that institution for that service. As a primary care provider, I was frequently thwarted by a patient or myself preferring a different locale for a service than contracted for by the patient's insurer. After awhile, when people expressed displeasure with their treatment options, I would recommend they change their insurer, as these decisions had been taken out of my hands. In fact, patients would often ask me which insurance to select when it came time for them to choose. I would generally recommend one that provided the largest, hassle free network. After all, I worked in Boston. There was no need to limit myself or my patients when the best in the world could be right next door, but inaccessible as far as my patient's insurance was concerned. The most audacious example of insurers contracting for specialty services was in the late 1980s, when the state of Massachusetts required insurers to offer *in vitro* fertilization services. One of the large HMOs in the state contracted with a group who had never had a successful pregnancy despite the fact that there were many more established groups in Boston who were quite good at the procedure. The high out of pocket cost of *in vitro* fertilization made the successful programs essentially off limits to my patients with the inferior HMO's insurance.

Having enough money to keep a health resource afloat may not always be easy. However, giving advantages to large health care organizations that focus on and support a corporate structure, has not worked well in my experience.

Chapter 7

Are HMOs the problem?

HMOs (Health Maintenance Organizations) have become the bad guys of health care. They were the alleged culprits who prevented us from doing what our patients needed, or who made us comply with silly documentation requirements. Indeed, I have filled out many a form to get a test or medication approved for a patient. However, I can not recall a necessary test ever being denied by an HMO. Of course they have denied tests such as neuropsychological testing (a detailed battery of cognitive tests used to assess brain function), requiring me to send the patient to a psychiatrist for an evaluation first, but this was a matter of style, and not substance. Neuropsychological testing was expensive, and if they could eliminate one test without a clear purpose, they could pay for 5 evaluations by psychiatrists. So, clearly the psychiatric evaluation was less expensive, and not necessarily, an irrelevant barrier.

I believe HMOs are the focus of our malcontent, but not the cause. HMOs extended health care coverage much further than it ever went before. When I was in med school in the early 1980s, a person's health insurance only covered sick care. Insurance companies didn't develop coding procedures for preventive health care visits until the early 1990s. If a doctor billed an insurance company service code for a sick visit and matched it with a patient diagnosis code saying the patient was healthy, the insurance company would reject the claim and not pay for the service provided. This left a doctor with the option of writing off the bill, or charging the patient, and have them complain that it should be covered by their insurance. Often a patient would ask me to modify the diagnosis on the claim so the insurance company would cover it (e.g. instead of saying a patient was completely health, I would use a diagnosis for a sore elbow, hay fever or some other benign condition). Of course, this led doctors to automatically bill for visits as though they were sick visits, to avoid such financial conflicts with their patients. Once the coding for preventive visits became standardized in 1992, annual physicals become routinely covered by HMOs, and we could finally use healthy as a "diagnosis" for our patients.

HMOs also lowered the cost of co-pays, making the concept of a deductible and 80/20 (where an insurance company paid 80% of a service, and the patient paid 20%) largely a thing of the past. This made visits affordable, and with the extension of this concept to medications, they also became more affordable. In some cases, HMOs had placed restrictions on access to care. However, in my experience, they had been reasonable, though at times, burdensome. I believed it was appropriate to ask physicians to justify their reasoning, at times, especially when the care ordered was expensive, or outside the normal pattern of care.

My sense is that HMOs, in large part, have broadened access to care by making routine care more affordable to patients. At times, HMOs have created obstacles for physicians when they have provided care for their patients. Yet, these obstacles aren't limited to just HMOs, but are part and parcel of all health insurers. The problem is not so much the limitations. Even Medicare, the non-HMO, governmental, health insurance program for senior citizens, has as many rules and restrictions as any HMO (e.g. essentially all insurers have lists of medications that require prior authorization on their part before a prescription written by a doctor is paid for by the insurance company). From my perspective, the major issue is the need for a standardization of rules, so providers can learn them once, and learn them well. During my latter years of practice, I had a dozen "playbooks" to follow as I cared for my patients. Each playbook was a manual distributed by each insurance company I contracted with, detailing their rules and regulations. This was a major obstacle when it came to providing efficient care. It also required doctor's offices, clinics, etc. to have additional personnel to help navigate and adhere to the myriad rules and regulations, so the doctors could do what they did best, see patients (which was code language for generate revenue).

A single set of rules would have been helpful, and need not have been linked to a single payer system. In fact, one of the more important reforms proposed by President Clinton in 1992 would have achieved this by standardizing a basic benefits package. However, he didn't have the political savvy to negotiate Washington Politics at the time, and thus, he was chewed up and spit out by the lobbyists. The day Hillary Clinton testified to the U.S. Senate with her initial presentation of the Clinton health care reform legislation, she was extolled as a great communicator and a formidable negotiator. In reality, the U.S. Congress was just setting her up for the inevitable fall they knew she would ultimately take. She came to epitomize the failure of the Clinton Administration to develop support for his health care legislation, which wasn't in the interest of the Congress or its contributing supporters (i.e. the health care and drug industries).

Thus, many of the ideas they proposed then never got off the ground. The well-defined benefits package they sought to develop would have prevented health care insurers from offering a package with little cost, but also, few, if any, benefits. All basic elements of care would have been required by all health insurance plans. A basic level of benefits would also have made it easier for people to compare insurance plans when deciding on a health insurer. People would no longer have to try to understand the fine print, or use a complicated spread sheet to project their costs when comparing plan A to plan B.

In addition to defining the basics of coverage (and thus, rules for obtaining that coverage), the Clinton plan also would have created health insurance buying cooperatives in each state. As a result, if a person's employer didn't offer a particular insurance plan, one could have opted out and purchased the insurance plan at a group rate from the state's buying cooperative. This type of system would have truly leveled the playing field. However, like most free market solutions to health care, those which permitted real, competitive forces were ignored, while those which touted a market solution, in reality, were not governed by free market forces.

Finally, the Clinton health care plan called for the establishment of a set of practice guidelines. Such guidelines would have created a set of rules governing how particular medical conditions were treated, which in the end, would likely have been a mixed blessing. If a practitioner followed these guidelines, and a patient had a bad outcome (e.g. they died unexpectedly), the practitioner would have been protected against a malpractice suit. Such guidelines gave the appearance of a suggested mode of treatment, yet ultimately, they could have become a constricting cookbook that limited assimilation of new and/or alternative information. Since such guidelines would have been defined by national consensus, they would inevitably have been a year or two out of date from current research. If one tried to stay at the forefront of managing a problem, one would likely be practicing outside of such guidelines, due to the inherent time lag between new data coming out, and the guidelines being updated. As a result, the guidelines would not only have given a practitioner tort protection, but conversely, if a practitioner didn't follow the guidelines, they could be vulnerable to malpractice claims. If a patient experienced a bad outcome (e.g. permanent nerve damage), even if the bad outcome was due to a well known, but rare, and thus, infrequently discussed side effect of a particular treatment, a practitioner not following the guidelines might be deemed liable for the bad outcome.

Practice guidelines also would have been inherently biased by the information structure that existed in Medicine. Evidence based medicine is the in vogue parlance for practicing Medicine using the medical literature as one's guide. In essence we all did this, though some, more closely than others. Unfortunately, much of what a primary care doctor sees on a daily basis hasn't been well studied due to the low mortality associated with these conditions (e.g. muscle spasm may cause disabling pain but you won't die from it). As a result, a practitioner has to interpolate from the medical literature on a daily basis. Guidelines could have made it hard to bring in alternative therapies, or even nutritional information, because much of what was known in those areas was not at the detailed level as the treatments of asthma and coronary heart disease (these are two diseases with an extensive medical literature defining their cause, and outlining effective therapy for them).

An example of a disorder in which there is disparity between the symptoms a patient might have brought to a visit, and the clinical diagnosis, is celiac disease (also known as gluten sensitivity or gluten enteropathy). It has become apparent that the spectrum of symptoms due to celiac disease may be much broader than just abnormal intestinal function. However, if a patient has a negative biopsy (i.e. no disease evident by microscopic examination of the biopsied tissue) of their small intestine (the gold standard for diagnosis in the eyes of a gastroenterologist), but has lab features suggestive of celiac disease, and symptoms that may be attributed to it, a trial of a gluten free diet is worthwhile. A gluten free diet is totally nontoxic therapy, but potentially requires a major life style change for the patient. Generally such a disorder is considered only when a patient has struggled with symptoms for years, and neither a specific diagnosis, nor effective therapy has been established by the patient or their physician(s). Thus, practice guidelines in an area such as this, where the spectrum of illness is still being defined and debated in the literature, could be problematic, and ultimately, stifling of practical or innovative care.

Indeed, HMOs aren't the cause of all health care problems, nor the major reason physicians are aborting their health care careers. Other contributing factors are the corporate approach to Medicine, drug companies and their high profit margins, the disparity in physician salaries, and the inability of physicians to be able to trade off part of their income for a style of practice more conducive to their needs and the needs of their patients. The major problem with health insurers, from my perspective, was the limitless rules and guidelines specified by each of the many insurers a physician had to deal with in order to support a practice. Thus, the most important need in this respect was a single set of rules for the basic issues a primary care practitioner dealt with 95% of the time. We need rules and regulations that won't change from insurer to insurer, and from day to day.

Chapter 8

Drug Companies

The cost of bringing a drug to market has often been quoted as $500 million. The $500 million figure came from a 1991 study by Joseph DiMasi of the Tufts Center for the Study of Drug Development which included every conceivable cost that could be attached to drug development. This skewed the figure upward, because much of the research and development (R&D) done by drug companies was not expensive, per se. In addition, the $500 million figure was inflated by including "lost income". This was income the drug companies claimed they would have earned had their R&D money been invested in Wall Street instead. Even when the drug companies did R&D, their cost for a "winner" (i.e. a drug that lead to enormous profits) could be a down right bargain. On July 23, 2001, the $500 million figure was challenged in a detailed and well documented analysis by Public Citizen (**http://www.citizen.org/congress/drugs/R&Dscarecard.html**). Their analysis supported a cost of $110 million for a drug company to bring a new drug to market.

An example of an inexpensive, but potentially financially rewarding drug development scheme involves the common phenomenon of making a copycat drug (referred to as a "me-too" drug in the Public Citizen report). When a successful drug had been brought to market for a novel indication (e.g. a drug to treat adult onset diabetes by making a patient's own insulin work better), the company who manufactured and supplied this drug would strike it rich. Since this type of drug therapy didn't previously exist, the new drug would have this niche all to itself. If it generated a lot of revenue, other drug companies would begin to focus their development on making a copycat drug. This copycat drug would be of similar structure and would work by the same mechanism as the original drug. Thus, this would be a relatively easy task, since the new drug's structure had already been published (in the medical literature and/or the patent application). An experienced organic chemist could study the structure of the original drug, and have a good idea how to modify it so that another drug like it would be sufficiently different to be patented, but still work in a manner similar to the original, novel drug. This process which netted significant revenue for all the major drug companies couldn't cost $500 million per drug; not even close.

In addition, modern molecular biology has simplified the screening and development of new drugs. At least once a month, I would read in *Science* magazine, a study published by a drug company which presented a new way to devise and/or screen for a new drug with a novel and likely very beneficial mechanism of action. Generally, I would read the details as to how they achieved their success, so I could get an idea of the cost involved. Using these state of the art techniques, I rarely could project even $1 million in development costs. Such studies were preliminary, and the cost of getting a novel drug through clinical trials would cost millions. Yet we would be talking about tens of millions to get there, not hundreds.

Finally, using modern day computing power and structural analysis of cellular receptors, drug companies could make excellent guesses about which chemical structures would be most likely to be successful. During the 1980s, when the cost data was generated to support the $500 million drug development figure, drug companies still used methods similar to those devised at the turn of the 19th century by German alchemists. Today, a drug company can get the published genetic sequence of a receptor and use a program to predict its structure, or even better, get an actual study showing the molecular structure of the receptor (often paid for with federal research funds). From this information, they could then guess which chemical groups would likely interact with this receptor, and do virtual testing on a computer before they would synthesize a single compound. They would still ultimately have to do bench top research to make the product, but substantially less research. As a result, the process has become less expensive, not more expensive.

You might ask yourself, why then are drugs so expensive? I have maintained that it is due to a need by drug companies to maintain stock value, and thus, sustain a particular level of return for the shareholder. Since all drug companies are in the same boat, they haven't undercut each other in price. As a result, the minor differences in price that competing drug companies charged had failed to lower appreciably the costs of medications. These practices sustain the revenues generated by those same drugs for the major pharmaceutical companies, and thereby, maintain their stock value. It might be easier to understand these factors, by looking at a specific example.

A new drug developed by drug company X would have a novel indication. Drug company X would enjoy no competition in the market for a year or two, until the first copycat drug came out by company Y. If drug company X needed to charge a patient $140 a month for their novel drug in order to cover costs, why did drug company Y need to charge $135? After all, the actual cost to company Y of making their copycat drug would have been substantially less than that of drug company X. In addition, drug company Y would want to get a significant market share with their new drug. This would not be any easy task, as once doctors became familiar with the novel drug of company X, they would be loathe to try the newer one due to the need to learn a new dosing schedule, potentially new side effects, etc. To counteract this barrier, why wouldn't drug company Y charge $70 (i.e. substantially undercut the competitor)? Drug company Y could still have made a handsome profit, developed a large market share, and would have had soaring sales, as it was likely all insurance companies would require doctors to prescribe the cheaper copycat drug. The insurance companies would assume the copy cat drug worked as well as the original product from drug company X, but cost them significantly less.

Competitive pricing has occurred in most other industries. During the Christmas season in 2000, I saw many copycats of the Razor® scooter. They weren't 5% cheaper than a Razor®, they were 50% cheaper. The drug example above used a 3% difference, which in my experience, was typical in the drug industry, not the 50% decrease, which was the type of behavior taught in business school.

In fact, I have never seen such discount pricing occur in the pharmaceutical industry during my 20 years in Medicine, and I would be surprised to see data to the contrary. In addition, I could generate countless examples of drug pricing similar to the one above. I would argue that drug company Y didn't undercut the drug price of company X because company X would have retaliated by lowering the cost of a drug of another class that competed with a company Y drug. This would have resulted in real price wars, and thus, the revenues of all drug companies would have plummeted. As revenues fell, stock prices would fall, and who would benefit then? Well, just about everyone who used a prescription medication. Who benefited by the current pricing system? Only the drug companies and their share holders did (look at major drug company stock prices in the 1990s). The anti-competitive pricing practices of pharmaceutical companies were unlike anything I had ever seen in any other industry. Airline companies were constantly having to defend against price fixing complaints. Yet their pricing practices were on a scale that paled in comparison with that done by drug companies.

We have permitted the pharmaceutical industry to hide behind third party payers, as most people who use expensive medications don't directly pay for them. In addition, when I served on the Pharmacy Committee of the academic medical center where I worked, I learned about rebates that the health insurance companies received from drug companies. The rebates were given in exchange for inclusion in an insurance company's drug formulary. A formulary refers to a specified listing of medications used by an institution (e.g. hospital, clinic or insurance company) to limit the choices of medication available from a particular class of medication (e.g. having only two of nine cholesterol lowering medications available). Formularies were first used for valid reasons by hospitals, who would make reasoned attempts to use cost effective and safe drugs. Insurance companies attempted to do the same, but the process has become so distorted by rebates, that it often made no sense to a physician why the insurance company selected a particular drug as their preferred agent for a specific condition. I often read reviews of new medications in the "Medical Letter" (a newsletter about medications, new and old, which includes their uses and costs). The "Medical Letter" generally lists the average wholesale price (AWP) of a 30 day supply of a common dosage of a drug they review. However, these prices were meaningless when I tried to decide what was cost effective for my patients. My patients' insurance company defined their formulary selections based on their cost, which could be substantially altered by rebates (some insurance companies would receive rebates totaling tens of millions of dollars per year from pharmaceutical companies). Even if the wholesale price of a drug I prescribed was less than the insurance company's formulary choice, my patient might incur a higher copay because I was prescribing a non-formulary medication.

Thus, the drug formularies of insurance companies only complicated the practice of Medicine. In addition, they effectively took prescribing decisions out of the hands of physicians. Every year I would get a new formulary from each insurance company for which I was a provider (about a dozen). They each sent me a letter telling me how important it was that I read the formulary and prescribed according to it. Frankly, I didn't have time to indulge their corrupt practices. I prescribed what worked for my patients, taking into account efficacy, side effects and other drugs they were taking. The only practical way to define a drug as cost effective was to use the AWP. I didn't have time to memorize the choices made by each insurer, nor did I have time to match each patient's insurance to the associated formulary book. When a health insurance company considered my prescription for a non-formulary drug sufficient to warrant a letter, I would answer them. Yet, to follow their formulary guide as though it were a bible, when it changed from year to year depending on whether the rebate they were offered from a drug company was sufficient to have their products listed on the insurance's formulary made no sense to me. A drug which the insurance company considered taboo one year could be in vogue the subsequent year.

A recent example of this phenomenon has occurred with the cholesterol lowering medication class referred to as "statins". In 1997, Zocor was clearly the most effective agent. I felt it was arrogantly priced by Merck as the most expensive in its class, despite its newness to the market (generally the new drug on the block is priced slightly less to try and gain market share). When Lipitor came out in 1998, Merck dropped the price of Zocor just below that of Lipitor. They then rebated their way on to most insurance company formularies. Despite a newer more effective agent being available (Lipitor), I was required to prescribe Zocor for many of my patients. This year (2001) it has all changed. Now, many of these same insurance companies have been asking me to change my patients taking Zocor to Lipitor. Didn't they think I had anything better to do than play their formulary games?

Chapter 9

Corporate Medicine II

In the mid to late-1990s, mergers weren't confined just to Wall Street. The rage had spread to the health care industry. Hospitals in the Boston area began to merge. The first shocker was Brigham and Women's Hospital (BWH) with Massachusetts General Hospital (MGH), both large hospitals affiliated with Harvard Medical School. Then, the two sister institutions at Boston University (BU), Boston City Hospital (BCH) and University Hospital (UH) merged. Finally, Beth Israel Hospital (BIH) and New England Deaconess Hospital (NEDH) merged. Prior to their merger, NEDH had been consuming many of the smaller community hospitals in the Boston area.

During the merger mania on Wall Street in the late 1990s, it was noted that the benefits to the consumer weren't always clear. Indeed, this lack of benefit to the consumer was definitely the case in the hospital mergers noted above. Just as on Wall Street, these hospital mergers were driven by a corporate mentality. Those managing the hospitals believed they had to be bigger if they were going to compete in the future. It seemed to be predicated on the assumption that if they weren't growing they were dying. At a minimum, the mergers further consolidated the hold that corporate medicine had on our nation's health care.

The major problem I saw with corporate medicine was that all services and care could be defined as interchangeable units. It didn't really matter who provided the service, if it was a 99213 (the billing code used for a basic office visit), it could be a nurse practitioner, a recently trained resident, or a highly skilled and experienced physician. Clearly the service provided by these three practitioners could be quite different. However, in corporate medicine, they were all viewed as the same, and thus, equivalent because they generated the same amount of revenue. In this model, skills were not considered an asset. In fact, this model preferred providers who could provide the service in the most cost effective way. The trick was to maintain a positive image of care at the institution, so that patients would remain interested in receiving their medical care there, even though it was offered by less experienced (and less expensive) personnel. Experience and a broad range of skills could actually become counterproductive from a manager's point of view. No frills, no deviations, the goal was to get the patients in and out.

All the hospital mergers noted above involved academic medical centers (AMCs). AMCs have been the hallowed institutions where innovations in health care were allegedly created. The AMCs had begun to sell their names not only as a way to draw patients, but ultimately to provide a vast network of clinics that could feed the parent hospital where the high tech and high cost procedures were done. The BWH and MGH merger, referred to as Partners, created a clinic in a flourishing western suburb of Boston, which they refer to in their ads as Mass General West. The only thing this clinic had in common with MGH was that they were owned by the same parent corporation (Partners). Often such centers were staffed by recently trained graduates who found the starting salary the most money they had ever made in their life (which wasn't hard since your maximum salary as a resident is about $40,000).

This type of satellite clinic would be smaller in comparison to a clinic in town, and thus, more personable. The corporation would have specialists come out periodically to support the generalist's care, but again, they were generally the lower ranking ones. While they could be fine physicians, they weren't the ones of the caliber used to generate the reputation of MGH, nor the ones who would continue to carry the day at MGH.

The AMCs hadn't limited the selling of their names to satellite clinics. They had also increased their financial relationships with biotech and drug companies. The AMCs were created in the mid-1960s as part of the

Medicare program. They were to foster research in patient care which would be used to advance the US health care system. Funds from Medicare were made available to train residents, so that hospitals wouldn't have to shoulder the training burden. In addition, the types of procedures done at some of these AMCs were quite involved, and required a higher rate of reimbursement than the usual care Medicare supported.

These were indeed noble goals. But just as the military industrial complex became the lobbying monstrosity that President Eisenhower warned us about, the AMCs had achieved a similar position in the health care industry. They had become so large in terms of the volume of money flowing through them annually, that they were a potent lobbying force. The most recent lobbying focus of the AMCs had been to get some of the federal budget surplus to compensate for the revenues lost during the Balanced Budget Agreement of 1997. The cash flow in health care had become so great, that the institution where I worked had a half billion dollars move through it each year by the late 1990s.

Yet, the most lucrative and potentially corrupt practice involving the AMCs has surrounded the indirect costs of government supported research. Indirect costs refers to an amount given in a federal research grant (usually from the National Institutes of Health, NIH) to develop and support the university infrastructure. Thus, when one obtained a federal research grant, he or she would have available a set amount of money (e.g. $1 million dollars over 3 years) which was to be used to cover the direct cost of the research. This would include not only project costs, supplies and equipment, but also salary support. In **addition** to this, the university who sponsored the researcher, would get 50-80% of the grant amount. It is important to understand that this was in addition to the amount already allocated as direct research costs (thus, the total cost to the NIH for a $1 million dollar grant would be $1.5-1.8 million over the three years).

The amount an institution received for indirect costs would depend on the standard amount they had been given in the past. There was essentially a formula used to define the base amount given to cover indirect costs (about 50%). However, universities that had created a large research infrastructure in an expensive part of the country (e.g. the Northeast and California) would receive more than the 50% baseline for indirect costs, at times as high as 80%. This money has been a major boon to the growth of the AMC. In fact, in the past decade at Boston University, I have watched three large research buildings constructed. The revenues for indirect costs were used to build this additional research space. These new facilities were used to attract more researchers who could get grants which would further add to the indirect cost revenues.

In the early 1990s, indirect costs of federal grants became a significant news item. At the time, the President at Stanford University, Donald Kennedy, had been using a yacht to entertain. The yacht had been used as a basis to inflate indirect costs. This and other extravagant expenses put indirect costs up for review. A group of accountants from the Navy looked into the Stanford scandal and similar issues at other universities. However, not much happened except for some "mea culpas" with small amounts of money given back to the government.

During the Clinton years, the NIH had its funding nearly doubled, going from about 12 billion when he came into office, with a projected budget of about 24 billion by 2003. Unlike the budget crunching days of the early 1990s, the NIH has been awash in money. Thus, there has been little concern of late about indirect costs. Yet these very dollars have helped to tilt the tables of health care to the AMCs. Many community hospitals closed in the 1990s due to tight Medicare and Medicaid reimbursements. The remaining community hospitals latched onto corporations dominated by the AMCs, which have had a major part of their infrastructure subsidized by the federal government.

The AMCs have not only benefited from facility fees, as I noted in the first chapter on corporate medicine, and their indirect cost subsidy, but finally, they have also benefited from the academic aura of seeking the greater truth, solely to provide the best in health care. Most AMCs have had both a clinical and research component. The research component has been most valued by management because of the revenues generated by indirect costs. A physician who got his or her grant funded would be able to stay in academic medicine. Those who didn't were asked to leave. If a physician researcher was also a clinician (i.e. he or she took care of patients), even a good one, he/she may not have been able to stay without a grant to support their salary. Most AMCs have developed a primary care practice in their clinics. This was done to increase the volume of primary care patients needed to feed the AMC's specialty practices. Thus, the AMC graciously have taken on a few layers of retail docs (primary care providers), to keep the patients coming.

Patients who have received their primary care at an AMC often have done so at greater expense to themselves. They would likely have had to pay for parking, which may well have been free at their local hospital. They may have had a higher copay from their health insurer, as health insurers generally charged more for a visit to a clinic than to a private office. In part, the higher clinic copay was created to offset the facility fee paid by the insurer to the AMC clinic. The facility fee also may have only been partially covered (e.g. Medicare recipient's would be required to pay 20% of the facility fee in addition to 20% of the doctor's fee). Many people would have put up with this either because they liked their provider, or they perceived added value in getting their care at an AMC. Visits with these patients have been the sole source of revenue for the primary care provider (i.e. primary care doctors only generate revenue by taking care of people, as they rarely do procedures). Yet these same patients have also served as fodder for the rest of the system.

The AMC was fed in part when the primary care provider referred a patient to have a test done. Of course, this was true of all hospitals. Hospitals generated revenue by providing not only laboratory services and x-rays, but also slightly more sophisticated tests like an echocardiogram (a test that uses ultrasound energy to take pictures of the heart). I was taken aback in 1996, when a patient of mine showed me a bill his insurance company had paid for an echocardiogram. They had paid $2000 for this test; $500 for the 5-10 minutes it took the cardiologist to read it, and $1500 to the hospital for providing the service and the facility (i.e. a place to perform the test). This type of test should have cost a few hundred dollars at most, if we had a fair and equitable health care system. Even if it took a cardiologist 15 minutes to read an echocardiogram, at $100 per test, he/she would make $400/hr. This would be well in excess of the hourly rate needed to pay a cardiologist an annual salary of $150,000 to 200,000. There was also no logical reason for the hospital to be paid more than $250 for providing a test which took about 1/2 hour to perform, and used technology which had been ripe for over a decade.

Fortunately for the AMCs, the clinical activities that generated the big dollars I alluded to in the "Welcome to Corporate Medicine" chapter, merged nicely with their academic mission. As the AMCs have done research to uncover effective, new procedures (usually through grants from the federal government, discussed in the Public Citizen Report at **http://www.citizen.org/congress/drugs/R&Dscarecard.html**), they have had a captive audience to which they could sell them. How much they should have been compensated wasn't easy to calculate, but it started to remind me of what the drug companies had done to exaggerate their developmental costs. Yet the federal government has been shouldering the cost burden ever since the AMCs were created as part of the Medicare legislation in 1965 (the NIH had been shouldering the grant burden since World War II). The AMC has not been able to see the forest, only the trees. They have consistently tried to log the best trees without consideration of the greater health care forest (like any good corporation would do). Every week I would have patients remark that their common ailments must have an effective therapy. They would hear news on a daily basis extolling the many advances in Medicine. Yet, they didn't realize that the news reports only talked about the prize catch. The rest of the ocean was depleted of stock and lacking in vitality.

Chapter 10

The Bean Counters

Documentation, documentation, documentation, was the mantra of the bean counters. After all, they were the ones who reviewed our office notes, and decided if the notes matched the billing codes we used for our office visits. One might think doctors would be careful in their documentation so that if they were sued, they could adequately defend themselves. This rationale was far from the case. Doctors documented according to standards set largely by the American Medical Association (AMA). The AMA developed a standard for coding services (Comprehensive Procedure Terminology, CPT). The fourth and current version, CPT-4 was released in 1992. This version was supposed to help physicians because it took into account the time and complexity of the care doctors provided. It also codified a documentation standard for reimbursement, which has been subsequently used by the bean counters to determine if the level of service we have billed has been adequately supported by our documentation in the office record (i.e. a patient's chart).

The standards in CPT-4 were quite simply written, and thus, could be broadly interpreted. However, to interpret them accurately, one would need to be a physician, as an untrained person couldn't discern whether a documented service met the medical complexity standards of CPT-4, or if the medical reasoning required to arrive at an assessment and plan of care was straight forward or not (this was another coding variable in CPT-4). Yet, such a monitoring system would be too expensive. An insurance company couldn't afford to use MDs to audit claims to see if the documentation (and thus, the level of service provided) warranted the charge

submitted. To avoid incurring such a cost insurance companies and corporate medicine devised another plan.

The clever answer of health insurers, which of course was endorsed by
the fiscally conservative AMA (of which I have proudly never been a
member), was to divide a typical office note into its component parts.
Then the bean counters could use a relatively simple formula to count up
the documented components, and translated this into a procedure code
for the service provided. This might sound simple, but it was dauntingly
complicated. This complexity of coding was not a trivial matter, but it was
assumed that if you could count beans, you could count up the number of
components documented in a note, and match it to a list that defined the
appropriate billing code. Unfortunately, these documentation requirements have left countless clinicians spending ever increasing amounts of
time documenting what they did. This in turn added to the difficulty of
making time to actually talk to a patient during a visit, and thus, ensure
that their issues were adequately covered.

The dogma of the bean counters was, "If it wasn't documented in the
chart it didn't occur" (and thus, couldn't be billed for, even if the service
was actually rendered). Think about the implications of this. How effectively can you remember the nuances of your work day, such that after a 4
hour period, you could write down sufficient detail that included minor
comments you made 2-3 hours ago? Furthermore, noting (in the patient's
chart) a comment made hours earlier, could determine whether you were
paid $50 for the visit or $75. The value the customer (patient) received
wasn't affected by this, only your reimbursement. The care you provided a
patient was completed with respect to the service you billed for when they
left your office, however, your worth financially was based on how well
you wrote it down afterwards. And this of course was the bottom line of
the bean counters.

In reality, one could bill any level of service (i.e. code) one would like.
However, the insurance companies had computer programs that identified
billing practices that tended to "over bill" (that is, exceed the average level

of service billed based on your specialty, location, etc.) Complicated stuff, eh? A health insurance company might consider a pattern of over billing if a practitioner consistently billed at the highest level of service, while the diagnoses used to justify the service were too trivial to support such extensive evaluations (e.g. a complete physical billed for every common cold seen in the office). After all, when a provider agrees to accept reimbursement from a health insurance company, he or she also agrees to their right to audit the records of their patients at any time. The health insurance company could decide after the fact, whether the documentation met the standards that currently existed (and not necessarily the standards that existed when one wrote his or her office note). This latter issue was a real concern, as Medicare had used the FBI in the late 1990s to investigate the billing practices of several AMCs. They used documentation standards developed in the 1990s to evaluate the adequacy of visits documented 1-2 decades earlier when documentation standards were rudimentary at best.

Medicine has a long tradition which has fostered predictability. This stability would be attractive to physicians who were risk aversive, and who wouldn't want to take a chance with something like documentation. One's inclination might be to exhaustively document patient visits to minimize the likelihood that an insurer would need to be paid back in the event a future audit suggested overcharging. The toll this takes on a practitioner who sees dozens of patients daily isn't trivial. A practitioner has at least 5-10 minutes of paperwork per patient visit. This time required just to write office notes, with the primary focus of the notes to meet the standards of third party payers (i.e. insurance companies). These documentation requirements didn't mean that the notes had more relevant information, or would help save a life. In fact, they often led to inordinate cluttering of information so the provider could be sure to include all points relevant to the billed level of service (i.e. trying to list as many of the billing components counted by the bean counters as possible). I would spend the equivalent of an eight hour day documenting my office visits each week. These eight hours didn't include time I used for documenting phone calls, nor letters I sent to patients, nor the development of additional treatment plans based on data received after a patient's visit.

This time commitment of documentation was exasperating, and served no purpose to benefit the patient, the doctor, nor the office staff. It only helped insurers decide if the incredibly low amounts they paid us for providing primary care were justified. One of the more distressing elements of this story has been the assimilation of these documentation practices by the physician leaders at major medical centers. The Chief of Medicine at my institution actually created a Compliance Office shortly after taking control in the mid-1990s. The people in the Compliance Office were to monitor our documentation to make sure it met third party standards. It was as though Big Brother had moved in next door. In addition, inordinate amounts of time were spent at our business meetings talking about the nuances of coding a visit for optimal reimbursement. The leaders have taken to groveling for every dollar they can get from insurance companies. The impact of this mentality, and the toll it took on the medical staff seemed to be viewed as inconsequential, but in reality was substantial.

Another aspect of documentation that was particularly bothersome to me was that no such standards existed for many non-clinical medical specialties. Radiologists, for example, had no standard way of documenting their interpretation of a chest x-ray. An x-ray report could state, "no interval change since the prior examination of (the prior date)". This type of information was not only not helpful, but provided no objective evidence that the x-ray had been adequately evaluated. Why in primary care was it assumed that it didn't happen if it wasn't written down, whereas radiologists could omit all relevant detail, and we were supposed to assume it was read thoroughly and correctly. Not infrequently, I had to look at an x-ray myself to make sure the specific question I had asked was answered, as the radiologist hadn't addressed it in the written report (e.g. a report of a shoulder x-ray stating there was no fracture of dislocation, but my question was, "Was there any arthritis?"). If standards did exist for the required elements in an x-ray report, they were not routinely implemented. I do not suggest that we should ask insurers to create an onus similar to that on primary care providers for radiologists also. I only wanted to stress the burden of documentation on primary care providers, and that similar documentation requirements did not exist across the board.

Standards and minimum requirements of documentation could be useful, but excessive detail required to facilitate monitoring of primary care services made no sense at all. There are times when a physician orders a test, but due to unexpected factors, the information resulting from the performed test is quite limited. A common example is an echocardiogram of a very overweight person. Changes in the chest wall due to the obesity prevent accurate measurement of some heart chambers. Thus, the effort required by the cardiologist to document the test result is less than expected, because only limited information resulted from the test. In such a case, the billing should reflect the deficient status of the data, and thus, the limited ability to make an interpretation. What I observed in such a case was a one paragraph echocardiogram report noting limited data, yet it was billed and compensated the same as one that comprehensively assessed all aspects of heart structure and function.

Office visit documentation requirements need to be lessened. As a quid pro quo, physicians would have a responsibility to not charge excessive amounts for simple, easy-to-provide services (there are some things that are easy to do which pay well, such as giving anti-inflammatory injections). Yet if anything, documentation practices have worsened. I received a notice from the Department of Health and Human Services dated 1 June 2000. It comes from Nancy-Ann Min DeParle, administrator at the Health Care Financing Administration (HCFA), the people who bring us Medicare. She notes, "Today I want to emphasize the importance of close attention to billing requirements, especially for documenting services delivered and the reason for care, as a way to ensure you receive and Medicare makes proper payments".

She added, "For physicians, we will be focusing this year on two CPT codes used to report evaluation and management services-99214 and

99233. These codes accounted for a significant portion of the coding errors in the last two audits. In fact, documentation for many of these services was only found to be sufficient to support services more appropriately described by CPT codes 99212 and 99231". To translate, 99214 refers to a CPT-4 billing code for a detailed office visit. CPT, as described above, was devised by the AMA and insurance companies to permit standardized billing by physicians and health care institutions. 99214 is sometimes called a level "4" service, as there were 5 potential codes used to bill an office visit with an established patient (defined as a person treated in the prior three years). 99214 is the fourth highest paying of the five visit codes. The memo implies that a number of claims billed at 99214 did not have adequate documentation to support that level of service (i.e. should have billed as a level 2 (99212) or level 3 (99213)). We don't really know if there was an excess of level 4 visits billed, as not documenting enough data points for the bean counters may have been the only problem. Yet even if there were cases of billing for a level 4 visit when a level 2 service was really rendered, it is a different issue (an office visit for level 2 would be a straightforward common cold in a young person, a level 4 visit would require assessment and documentation of at least two significant medical issues such as heart disease and diabetes). The amount of effort expended to perform and document a level 4 visit (30-40 minutes) was excessive.

A level five visit (99215) is used for complete examinations in patients who have multiple medical issues (e.g. congestive heart failure and diabetes). In the Boston area in 2000, Medicare paid $95 for such a visit. This type of visit requires at least 40 minutes with the patient, if not an hour, and another 10-15 minutes to write a note to document the service provided. This latter 10-15 minutes was the most important in terms of compensation, yet, the patient likely considered the first 40-60 minutes most important, as that was when the care was actually provided. However, the emphasis has been placed on what we document in that latter 10-15 minutes, as it determines how much we received and thus, our productivity.

At business meetings for the General Medicine Section of which I was part, we regularly discussed coding. We would review the myriad criteria used by us to decide the level of service (e.g. level 2, 3, 4 or 5) we were providing (and presumably documenting). People from the Compliance Office would review billing criteria with us to help us maximize our billing. Unfortunately, coding our visits had evolved into a game. It was hard to imagine some of the questions my fellow doctors would ask at these meetings. For example, "If I ask them (the patient) if their mother had diabetes, does that count as family history?", as family history gave a physician points with the bean counters when one tried to "maximize" their reimbursement.

The most perverse outcome of these billing requirements is the indirect incentive given to physicians to prescribe medication, with all their potential for side effects and cost, as opposed to using non-pharmacologic means. That is, we actually have incentives to prescribe a drug to treat a problem as opposed to using life-style modification, because it permits us to bill at a higher level. This is quite unfortunate, as there are multiple impediments to using life-style modification in clinical practice. The first disincentive was the time it took to educate the patient. The first step was to get the patient to agree that there was a problem that required therapy (this occurred when prescribing medications also). Then a physician would need to apprise the patient of their treatment options, and how to manage a life-style change. In addition, the physician needed to give the patient tools to accomplish and monitor a life-style change, setting specific goals (just as one might also do with medication). Yet the goals were not just numeric (e.g. lower the blood pressure under 140), but also behavioral (e.g. walk a total of 10 miles a week). People who had mild hypertension (high blood pressure) and were inactive, didn't just jump up off the couch and get moving. They needed specific direction on how much exercise to start with and realistic goals to accomplish before a return visit a month or two later. Patients also needed to learn how to avoid becoming overly enthusiastic, and end up with all or none behavior (e.g. either they were very good or very bad).

When faced with counseling a patient about a behavioral change to manage a problem versus prescribing a medication, one could bill based on time spent face to face with the patient. A clinician needs to spend at least 25 minutes discussing these issues to bill at a level 4 (99214) or 15 minutes face to face to bill a level 3 (99213). If a clinician spent 25 minutes talking to a patient, he or she would get $60-70 reimbursement from a third party payer for the 99214 you billed. Many physicians have found it more productive to see two level 3 (99213) patients during this 30 minutes (15 minutes on average per patient), and receive over $100 in compensation. However, each 15 minute visit meant in and out. There would be little to no time to discuss details such as what the patient was eating, what environmental factors could be contributing to his or her condition, and/or how the patient would become more active.

How does the physician keep the visit to 15 minutes and still treat the condition? The physician prescribes a medication. It is quicker, and for many conditions, it often works. Yet, if time alone wasn't enough incentive for a physician to prescribe a medication, the bean counters made it even better. When a provider prescribes a medication, the visit automatically rises from "low complexity" to "moderate complexity" (as discussed earlier, medical complexity is a billing component counted by the bean counters). The visit is considered low complexity when the clinician just talks about life-style modification. The levels of medical complexity established by CPT-4 are: straightforward, low, moderate and high. Straightforward implies that all physicians seeing such a particular clinical situation will in all likelihood arrive at only one outcome. (e.g. a person with decreased hearing due to wax in their ear; remove the wax and they will get better). A moderate complexity visit means if one's documentation is at level 3 in terms of historical information and physical exam (i.e. you have enough pieces of data in your note to satisfy the bean counters for a level 3 visit), the clinician may upgrade the coding to a level 4 visit just by prescribing a medication. However, if a physician does the same history and physical and decides that using the DASH diet (the standard diet for lowering blood pressure) should be the first approach in managing a person's blood pressure, the visit remains a level 3. Thus, prescribing a blood pressure medication in this case increases a physician's reimbursement for the visit by $15-20.

Documentation needs to be simplified so that primary care givers can record the core data needed to provide patient care. If we shift reimbursement to encourage physicians to talk to their patients by paying for time spent face to face, we can decrease the time spent documenting and learning about documenting, while enhancing the care we provide. This would require a major overhaul in current thinking. At the beginning of 2000, the Health Care Finance Administration (HCFA), who manages Medicare for the US Government, put on hold new documentation requirements, which had been established in collaboration with the AMA. Believe it or not, they were much more onerous than those I describe above (which surely weren't straightforward)! Thus, as with many things in health care, it doesn't appear we are heading in the right direction.

Chapter 11

Do we earn too much?

I tend to think that as a profession, we physicians are overpaid. Of course, if you ask any particular physician, he or she will tend to feel they are undervalued. My final income as a physician just topped $100,000 a year. I recognized this placed me in the top few percent of Americans, and I found this more than acceptable. In fact, I have made it clear to my boss in the past, and to the medical community at large in a letter I had published in the New England Journal of Medicine in 1998, that I was willing to make less money if it permitted me to practice Medicine in a way more conducive to my needs.

I was willing to earn less if it permitted me more time to talk to my patients. When I had ample time to explore the issues brought forth with each visit, I not only could do a better job, but I enjoyed it much more. In fact, on days when I was able to practice this way (due to cancellations and no shows), I actually left satisfied and refreshed. Thus I asked myself, why couldn't everyday (or at least most days) be like this? I was willing to make the sacrifice financially. After all, I was trained to practice Medicine, not to make a lot of money or to document in order to maximize billing. However, I have faced nothing but barriers when I tried to develop such a practice.

When I was in solo private practice, I was able to control the time aspect of my practice. However, concerns over capitation led me to a group and the corporate medical model. In the seven years since I left private practice, the corporate model has become even more the norm. A physician's ability to negotiate a style to meet his or her individual needs has become nearly impossible. When I discussed the time I needed to see patients with my boss, he felt that if he let me have longer appointments with patients, then others in my group would demand it. In addition, he felt they wouldn't be willing to take a commensurate cut in pay, as I was willing to do. I have found this rationale shallow and conservative to say the least. I didn't see how such a simple quid pro quo could be a problem for my colleagues, who were pretty good at complex reasoning.

Physician compensation wasn't just an issue of being willing to work for less money so one could improve one's work environment. If you looked at the average doctor salary, you would find it had grown close to $200,000 per year. So why was my salary so low in the first place, relative to the average? Who was making all the money? Simply stated, specialists have been driving much of the cost of health care. However, a critical analysis of this income disparity didn't make sense. A couple of examples would demonstrate the point.

A colleague of mine told me about a radiologist in the Boston area who was a contemporary of ours (i.e. early 40s). He had three years of post-graduate training (the time after med school), like the average general internist or family practitioner. Yet he earned $350,000 a year, and had 10 weeks of vacation. So what did this person do to deserve such an income? The answer was simple: he went into a field of Medicine that was over-reimbursed. Radiologists are paid for each x-ray they read. They often will bill for two tests related to a single procedure (e.g. a CAT scan of the abdomen may be billed as one of the abdomen and one of the pelvis if cuts (slices of an x-ray) are taken low enough down in the body). Their reimbursement isn't based on how many films you would expect the average radiologist to read in a day, but just on the actual readings. This is consistent with the philosophy that those who work harder will get ahead. However, if the average number of films a radiologist can read leads to a $200,000 annual salary, have they earned it? How dose their effort and training compare to a primary care practitioner who may earn half that amount?

Why does a person who has no more training in their specialty than a family practitioner (who, like an internist, has three years of post-graduate training) earn so much more money? They have different training, but that is expected. After all, they learn how to read x-rays, and we learn how to take care of people. Yet this difference in training should not distort the value placed on one type of physician over another! Unfortunately, this type of disparity has remained typical in Medicine, and not at all an exception. In fact, it is one of the main reasons that medical students are shying away from primary care once again (as in the late 1980s).

Five years ago I was visiting a friend of mine who was an anesthesiologist practicing in Georgia. As an anesthesiologist, his job was to give medications to people so that they could have surgery or other procedures, without undue pain or discomfort. Surely, this was important. However, he also had the typical three years of training after med school. Yet he felt that he would never accept less than $150,000 a year as starting compensation for work in his field. At the time of our discussion I wasn't even earning $100,000. I had double the post-graduate training (6 years) and had been out practicing for five years (he was just out of training).

This kind of thinking has not only inflated our perceived value of ourselves, but also has led to business school like decisions amongst trainees. In June of 2001, I saw a fourth year Boston University medical student for whom I had provided primary care. Her course in med school was slowed by a couple medical problems, which prolonged her stay. Partly as a result of that, she became interested in primary care. When we last talked in the winter of 2001, before the Residency Match, she was talking about a career in women's health. When I saw her in June, she was going to be starting at a local community hospital as a medical intern. However, instead of a career in women's health, she had changed to anesthesiology. I asked her the current starting salaries (i.e. for someone right out of anesthesiology training, 3-4 years total), and she told me they were $200-300,000 a year (at least my friend in Georgia would have had his needs met). In this case, the income disparity between anesthesiology and primary care had unequivocally affected her decision not to enter primary care, yet her empathy and understanding would have been valuable assets for patients. Her concern was med school debt (which would remain deferred in terms of payments until she completed her anesthesia training), which would have been nearly impossible to pay back over the 10 years they were due if she went into primary care.

Her need for a high salary to compensate for substantial med school debt could be argued effectively. However, some of the ways physicians have earned income has been downright bothersome. Early in my private practice days (the early 1990s), I was having a discussion with a med school classmate of mine who had completed an oncology (the treatment of cancer) fellowship after his internal medicine training. He was making enormous amounts of money (at that time over $300,000 a year). Since he didn't have much to speak of in terms of procedures (he could occasionally bill for a bone marrow biopsy, but this didn't generate a lot of income), I was perplexed by his earning power. I then learned that he had adopted a common practice amongst oncologists when he went into private practice. He would purchase the chemotherapy drugs to be given to his patients in an outpatient setting, and when they came in for a treatment, his nurse would administer them. Nothing unusual there. What was remarkable was the ability to mark up the chemotherapy drugs they were purchasing on behalf of their patients. In addition, they could have a nurse give the drugs, and bill another $30-40 for each patient to whom they administered the medications. When a single nurse gave therapy to 30-40 patients a day, it would really add up.

I would wager the oncologist might argue that these drugs needed great care when administered (indeed some did), and that the nurse needed to monitor patients after giving the drugs for side infects (as he or she indeed did need to do). But this amounted to a nurse generating over $1000 per day in revenue, with the nurse seeing little of it. The oncologists got the lion's share, and for what reason? That they were supervising the use of poisons in a controlled fashion (my overall view of oncology, the treatment of cancer)? This is not to argue that they were not due some compensation for this type of supervision, but as with the other examples above, compensation should be in proportion to the level of expertise required.

Attempts had been made in the past to try and equalize the playing field. In the early 1990s, a relative based valuation (RBRV, relative base relative value) system was proposed, and partially implemented. The problem was that some professions (e.g. radiology, ophthalmology and anesthesia) had created over billed profiles in the past, so that a 50% cut still amounted to maintaining notable disparities in the system. In the final chapter, I discuss some strategies that I think may be helpful in trying to remedy this situation. If we don't try to level the playing field, it will surely continue to affect the pool of new entrants into primary care medicine.

Chapter 12

What does experience get you?

I have become old enough to have learned the value of experience. In my younger days, pure youthful enthusiasm, and intelligence could keep me ahead of the pack. As I have had more opportunity to witness the ways of the world and Medicine, in particular, I have been able to gain a perspective that cannot be taught, but only slowly garnered. I have learned when to be patient, and when to "step on the gas". In addition, the sheer depth of my knowledge has increased beyond what I would ever have expected. I can still remember many things verbatim as they were taught to me in med school and during my residency. I also have been able to fine tune this knowledge with experience, which has taught me, just because it made sense, didn't mean it was true.

So what had this experienced gained me? A comfort level with my knowledge base, to be sure. It has led to colleagues asking my opinion as to how they might have managed a difficult clinical problem. It has given me the opportunity to share my clinical skills with my colleagues during Medical Grand Rounds (the big academic conference each week) and to teach medical students and internal medicine residents when I am supervising on the hospital wards. It has also given me a cadre of faithful patients, who implicitly trusted my judgment. It has also given my patients long waits between appointments, because my superiors desired to maintain a particular output (i.e. productivity). It has made it harder for me to talk with my patients, to find out what made them tick, and to understand their issues during the times allotted. It has made me feel rushed and at times, harried. In other words, in terms of what I did most of the time, i.e. take care of patients, it didn't have as many returns as I had hoped.

So, what was the point? To use a metaphor; when I played hockey in my 40s, I no longer had the legs on the ice (and some might argue I never did) to keep up with 20 year olds who skated alongside me. Yet I could see the ice and the play of the game much better now than during my youth. What I now lacked in speed, could partially be compensated for by my improved view of the play. Similarly, I didn't have the energy of the 25 year old residents I taught, but I could help them see the big picture, and keep the residents from barking up the wrong tree. My experience was at least partially compensated. I was able to precept residents in their primary care clinics, which afforded me the opportunity to help them develop a long term perspective when managing a patient's issues (as I would tell them, "you can't run a marathon in the first mile"). I was also asked to serve as ward attending, and share my knowledge and judgment with medical students and residents as they confronted and managed potentially seriously ill patients.

Yet, these activities were at best a quarter of my annual schedule. The bulk of my time was spent as a primary care doctor. I saw people, I listened to them, I evaluated their situation and I helped them devise a plan for managing their medical problems. What did my experience get me in this bulk of my work load? It definitely got me the multitude of problems I have already noted in earlier chapters. Yet, it didn't allow me more time to talk with people, which was my main pleasure in primary care (the intimate sharing of medical issues with patients allows us to experience some vicarious living). It didn't give me more time to explore areas of interest to me (both within Medicine and in other areas). It didn't give me more time with my family (just to keep up with paperwork, I found myself going in for 6 hours one Saturday per month). So what was the point (it surely didn't give me more money, though my boss kept giving me nominal annual raises hoping the crumbs would do the trick and keep me satisfied)?

A colleague of mine confided in me, that in 1996, his superior had thought of letting him go as a free agent, because he had fresh young faculty members ready to take his place. My colleague was a bright, hard working cardiologist. He had always taken the practice of cardiology seriously, understanding the complex nuances of cardiac disease. He was affable, and an outstanding teacher. But he wanted a raise. He could have doubled his salary by leaving for private practice. He likely would have left the academic medical center (AMC) if his boss didn't move up the ladder, clearing the way for a new chief of cardiology, who valued his clinical skills. He still could have earned double his current salary in private practice, but at the AMC he was able to obtain some respect for his activities, and some time to develop areas of interest to him. I'm sure this was only partial compensation, but enough to keep him on board for the time being.

As I alluded to earlier, this wasn't about making money. I felt that I made plenty of money. I noted earlier, even though I was on the low side of the doctor pay scale, my income still permitted me to be in the top 1% of American wage earners. The problem that I had was the inability of the health care system to distinguish one's work from another. The health care system reinforced filling in the boxes, and making the coding of services match up with one's narrative. If they matched, one was paid, if they didn't, one would take a pay cut. The amount one received when submitting a billing code was the same in one's first year as a practicing physician, as in one's twentieth year. I'm not aware of this extent of disregard for experience in other professions.

We have developed a system of health care that has encouraged the cheapest form of delivery, by the least experienced practitioner. There were some time management skills that practitioners needed to learn, but from a corporate point of view, all primary care providers were interchangeable. health care was at a stage equivalent to when the automotive industry was being converted to a production line. As in those times, the Health care system had people who were trying to analyze the minimum amount of time needed to perform service X, and making that the standard. It has been referred to as "productivity", but it has been much more destructive than productive.

Chapter 13

The Form Doctor

Some days, it seemed that the major task of the day was to complete forms. I felt as though I had become a "form doctor". One of the great things about primary care is that we get to fill out the forms. It isn't that specialists don't fill out forms. Sometimes they make disability assessments, or need to fill out insurance forms to justify a therapy within their specialty. But primary care doctors get all of them, every conceivable type. We got Visiting Nurse Association (VNA) forms, durable medical goods forms, transportation forms, disability forms, food pantry forms, housing forms, etc. If there was an interface between your patient and an outside provider or service, whether medical or not, you could be sure there was a form for you to complete associated with the service.

Some forms are perfunctory. The durable medical goods forms tend to be easy. Most often they come from a local company that generally rents, but occasionally sells, durable (as opposed to disposable) medical equipment. Common examples of durable medical goods include a commode, a walker, a booster for a toilet seat, etc. The forms for these items come with a generic request letter and an attached page with all of the information completed. Thus, I only had to review the information, decide if it was appropriate, sign it and put it in the pre-addressed envelope. These types of forms generally needed to be renewed annually.

Other forms require a bit more time. Many of these come from the VNA. It is the VNA who often provides patient information to the durable medical goods company about which supplies a patient needs. However, the major role of the VNA is to provide home services for elderly or infirmed patients after hospitalization. To get VNA services, a person needs to be home bound (i.e. physically incapable of leaving the home). At times, the VNA has to overstate the extent of a person's disability in order to be able to provide the services the patient needs. After the VNA's initial assessment, they send the primary care provider a 2-3 page form to review and sign. It lists all the medications (which are worth reviewing, as occasionally the list does contain an error), all the services provided, and great, exhaustive detail about any special nursing services that are provided (e.g. details about wound dressing changes). However, many of the VNA reports I received were redundant and did not add to the information already in a patient's chart. As forms went, the VNA reports were pretty easy to sign off in good conscience and return in the envelope provided.

One of my favorites involved forms which clearly stated that they were to be completed by the patient (i.e. the form would specifically state, "to be completed by patient"). It wasn't only patients who would ask me to complete their parts of the form, but also other providers. There were several forms from the state, which only required a health care professional (which could be a nurse, social worker, psychologist, physician, physical therapist, etc.) to complete the form. When I received a form to complete from a patient's social worker, when they also could have completed the same form themselves was frustrating, to say the least. Patients often treat jury duty forms in a similar fashion. Under our current legal system in Massachusetts, all adults get a jury duty form every three years. Some of my patients would decide they couldn't serve due to their medical condition, and send the form right off to me. They never bothered to read it (or have someone read it to them if they couldn't do so themselves), though it clearly required them to complete and sign it. I suspected that illiteracy and cultural differences might have contributed to some of these forms coming my way, but when they added to a growing pile of other forms to complete, it was difficult to be empathic.

Yet, the forms I dreaded most were medical disability forms. These were the most problematic because they had a lot of questions that needed to be answered, and they just kept coming, one after another, month after month. First I needed to define the condition causing the disability. Then I needed to note whether it met one of the categories accepted as a cause of disability, or it met disability standards, without meeting a specific disability criterion. Next I noted what my patient could and couldn't do. There were questions about how many hours my patient could sit per day (the range was 0-8 hours). After each question like this was another question about my patient's ability to sit if they had breaks as opposed to doing it continuously (i.e. sitting all day). There were similar questions about standing, bending, lifting (and how many pounds my patient could lift: 0-10, 10-20, 20-40, >50?). Finally I had to explain what I was doing about the problem, and how long the disability was likely to last.

The disability forms from the Commonwealth of Massachusetts and Social Security were different from those provided by insurance companies. The latter's forms were very interesting indeed. Not only were disability insurance company forms the most burdensome because of the rapidity with which they came, but they often contained questions that seemed to have an adversarial tone (e.g. if patient wasn't getting worse, why couldn't he or she go back to work?). They also often required a return to work date, even when my prior forms had indicated clearly that the person was totally and permanently disabled (this was the way disability lawyers liked me to write it).

The biggest problem with the disability forms was that doctors rarely received specific training in assessing disability. I began to teach residents in primary care clinic about occupational health, but I never had formal training in it myself. What I learned and taught was from experience and the limited published information I found in the general medical literature. Doctors are thrust by the legal system into a role which most of us are totally incapable of handling well. The other issue in this regard, especially with private disability insurance, is the roadblocks that are continually thrown in the way of people who are truly hurting (physically and emotionally). These barriers may take the form of continued requests for additional information or recurrent hearings required by the disability insurer.

The disability insurance industry has many attorneys on their staffs. They are able to constantly create obstacles that make it difficult for injured people to make a fair claim. At least once a year I had a patient who couldn't afford his or her medications because the disability insurer stopped their payments and thus, their source of income to pay for their medications. (Once a patient's condition is linked to a disability insurer, all health care payments related to that condition come from the disability insurer. If a person's disability award is due to headaches, the person's health insurer will not pay any health insurance claims that use headache as the diagnosis. All claims for service using headache as a diagnosis must go through the disability insurer, even if the claims are made decades later. Disability insurers appear to review their case files about once every three to five years. It seemed apparent to me that the disability insurers had rules about how many cases they needed to move off the rolls so as to maintain profitability. I imagined (rightly or wrongly) that the reviewers and attorneys had quotas about how many cases they would be expected to ax per unit time (i.e. there would be an expectation that they could remove a defined number of active disability cases from the rolls every month). Often my patients who transiently lost their disability status would be reinstated later, but not without undue stress, anguish and potentially without treatment during that time for their medical condition. In addition, patients frequently had to hire an attorney who specialized in disability law just to salvage their benefits.

The Social Security Administration (SSA), which has managed long term disability (SSDI, social security disability income) for the U.S. Government, was just as bad. In fact, I never saw an SSDI claim go through on the first application. It appeared to be automatically denied the first time around. I routinely had to counsel patients to reapply, as this was just 'part of the process'. My suspicions about the perfunctory first application rejection by SSA were confirmed when a patient of mine who was dying of gastric cancer was rejected. Prior to her cancer, she had provided customer assistance for over five years at a local department store.

She worked despite panic attacks that were difficult to control, hypertensive heart disease and sleep apnea. When she contracted stomach cancer, I convinced her to stop working and apply for disability. I even had to implore her to appeal her denial. I believe she received benefits for a month or two before she finally died.

If filling out forms wasn't sufficiently onerous, at times I had to write a letter just to obtain the form which needed to be completed. For example, if a patient needed to miss work due to a short term disability, there were two ways to begin the process. One was available to all, an unpaid leave of absence under the Family Medical Leave Act (initially vetoed by G. H. W. Bush, but signed into law in 1993 by President Clinton). The second was through a short-term disability application. Both methods had associated forms which were to be completed by a physician. Many workplaces required a doctor's letter stating that the employee was ill and needed time off. This led the employer to give the physician a form to complete which requested information identical to that included in the letter about the patient's disability. I couldn't just ask the employee to get the form, a letter was generally required.

The most distressing aspect of disability forms is that they never end. Even patients with chronic, progressive conditions need to have a form completed annually stating that they aren't getting better. At some level, I understand the rationale behind such a request, as insurers don't want to continue to pay if a claim is inactive. Yet I experienced such requests as another attempt to steal time from me. Over time, I felt required to keep copies of the forms I completed, so I could make sure every year's version was consistent with prior years. Any deviation from year to year in how I completed the form would be noted by the disability insurance company, and would lead to a letter or phone call that required a response from me. Thus, even more time would need to be devoted to disability issues.

At times I found myself advising patients about how to proceed with disability claims. In general I recommended that if lost wages weren't involved, and the only issue was an injury, they should manage it through their health insurance. I didn't recommend this just to avoid disability forms, though surely it was tempting. I did it because I had seen people not be able to get the care they needed for a medical problem due to delinquent disability payments. Despite the agreement made by the disability insurer and my patient over what illness was covered, and what would be compensated, sometimes the insurer would just stop paying for unclear reasons. Even in cases where a judge ruled against a disability insurer in favor of my patient, there was little if anything done to the disability insurer for non-payment. My patients would just accrue medical bills related to their problem, and hope that eventually the disability insurer would start to pay again. Recently, when a young patient of mine with a work-related knee injury requested an evaluation, I strongly recommended that he treat it as a strict health problem to be managed by his health insurance. Otherwise, he risked having his knee "carved out" of future health insurance policies as a pre-existing condition. This would require all treatment of that knee for the next 40-50 years of his life to be managed through the disability insurance company of the employer who handled the original claim rather than through his health insurance.

The final form of frustration was the unexpected one. This was often a letter requesting that I defend my actions. A recent example was a form I received related to a patient I admitted to the hospital for fevers, weakness and severe anemia. There was no obvious infection causing the fever, so he wasn't on antibiotics. He was able to eat well enough, so he didn't need an IV (intravenous line to give fluids and medicine). He was a Jehovah's Witness, so despite his severe anemia, and symptoms related to it, he wasn't going to be transfused blood due to his religious beliefs. Yet he was ill, had been unsuccessfully battling his disease as an outpatient, and there were still diagnostic uncertainties about the cause of his illness. While he was in the hospital, we got his blood pressure under control and did a couple diagnostic tests which weren't easy to obtain on an outpatient basis. After a couple days, he went home feeling better than when he entered the hospital.

Yet, because we didn't put an intravenous line (IV) in him, or place a tube into any orifice (e.g. mouth, bladder, etc.), he wasn't deemed appropriate for admission. I had to justify in a letter to the insurance company why I had the audacity to admit this man to the hospital. If he hadn't been a Jehovah's Witness, he would likely have been transfused, thus satisfying the health insurance company. Yet, his religious beliefs prevented this, and thus, he was deemed inappropriate for admission. I have had colleagues who gave patients IV fluid unnecessarily, just to medically justify their patient's hospitalization. Hospitals have become places where we do things to people (e.g. procedures and treatments). We no longer have the luxury of viewing hospitals as a place to care for the seriously ill, regardless of the specifics of their care. Most of the time the two coincide, those seriously ill need to have things done to them. When they don't, a doctor can well expect a letter asking why, and …please, answer in detail!

Recently, another example of the surprise type of letter involved a colleague of mine. She had cared for a young woman who felt feverish and fatigued. She did an extensive evaluation, including laboratory testing, trying to decipher her illness. She gave the patient instructions on how to manage her illness in the two week interval between the initial evaluation and her follow up visit. Yet, the patient felt it wasn't enough. She complained to her insurance company, who requested the doctor send them a letter detailing her justification for her treatment plan. This letter was in addition to the detailed office note she had already written about the services provided to the patient.

I realize that there are doctors out there ignoring patient complaints. In these cases, such a letter of justification may be appropriate. Yet the entitlement that some patients have come to expect from our health care system has been excessive. I found that people called with common maladies, which were best handled by rest and time, but that some patients demanded same day treatment, largely because it was covered by their health insurance (and often, they paid dearly for this insurance). A primary care doctor's ability to use his or her medical judgment was no longer relevant or possible. Responding to such patient and insurer requests became imperative, or Big Brother would take action against one (with the appropriate paper work, of course).

Chapter 14

What to do about Medicine?

In this book, I have been very critical of the health care system (HCS). I believe my criticism has been valid. Yet, I also believe that criticism should be followed by constructive recommendations. Toward that end, I would recommend the following changes to our HCS. Some of these would be more easily implemented then others. In fact, some would require a wholesale restructuring of the HCS.

The first change would indeed be fundamental. It would require the HCS to change fundamentally its reinforcement system. As Pavlov showed at the turn of the 20th century, reinforcement patterns are critical when trying to elicit and sustain a specific behavior. I feel it is imperative that the HCS reinforce the importance of doctors talking with their patients. It has often been stated to medical students that the history one obtained from a patient contained 80% of the information needed to make a specific diagnosis (some would have argued more than 80%, but not less). The only way to obtain a patient's medical history still requires talking to people. But, the HCS based reimbursement more on what was done to people, than the discussions doctors had with them.

Thus, a major restructuring to support doctors talking with their patients is needed. The only way to ensure this result would be to de-emphasize the lopsided reimbursement of procedures. This would likely be fought tooth and nail by the powers that be in the HCS, as they have accrued their power by manipulating our current, distorted system. Yet, if the people (the patients) speak loudly, clearly and consistently about having time to talk with their doctors, indeed it could happen.

In addition, this primary interaction, the face to face interaction between the doctor and the patient, would need to be elevated to the apex of our HCS pyramid. It would need to be reinforced financially (likely with a time based reimbursement system), and also widely available. Such a change of focus would make it easier for doctors to open up shop where the patients are, instead of being limited to the increasing confines of the corporate medical elite which benefit from subsidies (i.e. facility fees and indirect cost payments). Since talking to a patient would be considered the primary focus of the HCS in this model, a physician wouldn't feel rushed during a visit with a patient. Spending more time with the current patient would be just as financially advantageous as proceeding to the next one.

Ideally, the HCS would permit a primary care physician to be able to hang out a shingle, talk to patients, and obtain adequate reimbursement. This latter objective would be facilitated by a HCS that ensured low overhead. To lower the overhead of a medical practice, the HCS would need to agree upon a universal set of rules. Yet all rules would be beholden to the primary rule, that the face to face interaction of doctor and patient could not be undermined. Also, the HCS would need to support the efficiency and uniformity of process, to prevent an undue burden on physicians' time spent away from their patients.

Much of what President Clinton tried to do in 1992 would have improved the efficiency of the HCS, from a primary care provider's perspective. It may not have been the best way to do it, but unfortunately, a real discussion of the problems with the HCS never occurred. The health insurance industry feared real competition in the health care market. They had become fat cats in the current HCS, and wanted it to stay that way. They concocted the Harry and Louise ads to bring it home (i.e. defeat the bill in Congress), and that they did. Next to Clinton's impeachment, his failure to get health care reform through Congress at a time when reform was so broadly supported by the electorate, may be considered one of his greatest failings. The insurance buying cooperatives President Clinton wanted established in each state were sorely needed in 1992, and remain important today. They are a tool that would allow customers (patients) vote with their feet, and choose an insurer of their liking, as opposed to being forced to accept the insurer who gives their employer the cheapest policy rate.

In addition to discouraging a procedure first mentality in Medicine, equity in physician reimbursement remains an important issue. The salary disparity between physicians of equal training needs to be resolved. Of course under these revisions, those earning more revenue than at present would be happy and those receiving less would be upset. I believe this potential problem is manageable. As I alluded to earlier, most primary care physicians make adequate livings. What they really need is a restructuring of their work environment. Since this change could lower their productivity (i.e. how many patients they could see in a day), to maintain their salaries, the money would have to come from somewhere else. I would view the primary donors as: radiologists, anesthesiologists, ophthalmologists and possibly pathologists. The doctors in these specialties would be upset, and strongly oppose such a change. Yet, would their opposition be credible? After all, they don't necessarily have more training than a primary care doctor, only different training. Surgeons do require extra training (at least two more years) and should receive additional compensation for it. In addition, in order to ensure adequate numbers of specialists, there needs to be some incentives toward that end. These incentives need not be all financial, but they surely could be. When a specialty was showing signs of a shortage, reimbursement could be enhanced, or programs to pay back student loans for people entering those specialties could be established.

Finally, the HCS needs to recognize experience. Many people wouldn't want a rookie treating them, but our HCS could become the Montreal Expos of health care if we don't do something to show that experience is valued (i.e. the HCS could be fielding what is in effect a minor league team in the major leagues). Reimbursement needs to factor in years of experience, and other special training or skills that enhance the primary interaction of doctor and patient. This may include skills in nutritional or behavioral change counseling. Other procedural skills and training should be supported, but not at the expense of the primary, face to face interaction of doctor and patient.

There are other factors such as the cost of medicines which also should be reformed. After all, we are the only country in the world that doesn't regulate the wholesale costs of medications. These and other structural reforms, will be important, but I wanted to emphasize those which have impacted most upon my journey in Medicine.

Ultimately, meaningful reform will be a tall order for our HCS. Yet, to ignore the realities I have discussed in this book would be to our own detriment. I have not been alone in my departure from Medicine. In fact, most people who read these pages likely will have heard about other doctors leaving Medicine. If we, as a society, don't act to reform the current health care system so that it supports primary care, then we'll be left with this reality: "Medicine's a good 20 year profession".